Principles of
Child Care

Conception to Childhood

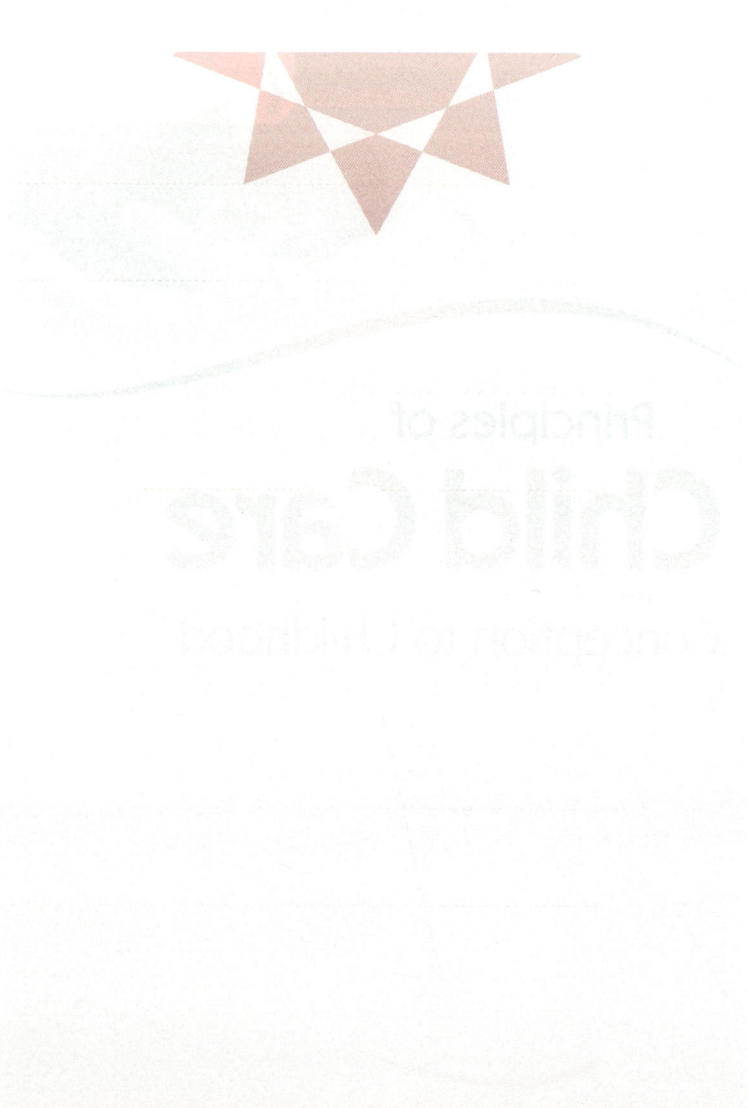

Principles of Child Care: Conception to Childhood
is a publication of the Health Care and Research Association for
Adolescents (Concept—Conception to Adolescence)

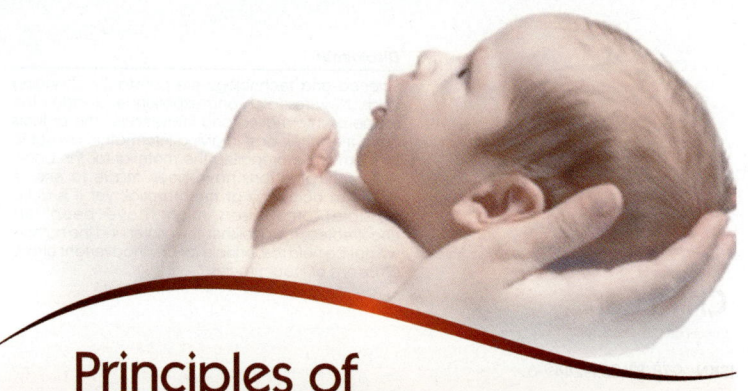

Principles of
Child Care
Conception to Childhood

KN Agarwal MBBS, DCH, MD, MD (Ped), FIAP, FAMS, FNA

Chairman, Pediatrics and Neonatology, Metro General Hospital, Noida, UP
Professor of Pediatrics, UCMS, Bhairwah, Nepal
Former : Faculty, Department of Pediatrics, Maulana Azad Medical College, New Delhi
Banaras Hindu University, Varanasi
University College of Medical Sciences, Delhi
Director, SGPGI Medical Sciences (Superspeciality Institute), Lucknow
Director/Dean, Institute of Medical Sciences, Banaras Hindu University, Varanasi

DK Agarwal MBBS, DCH, MD

Former: Pediatric faculty at Safdarjung Hospital, New Delhi, and
National Institute of Communicable Diseases, Delhi
Professor of Maternal–Child Health, Banaras Hindu University, Varanasi

CBS Publishers & Distributors Pvt Ltd

New Delhi • Bengaluru • Chennai • Kochi • Mumbai • Pune
Hyderabad • Kolkata • Nagpur • Patna • Vijayawada

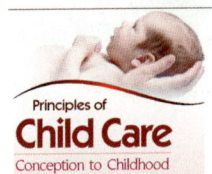

Principles of
Child Care
Conception to Childhood

ISBN: 978-81-239-2449-6

First Edition: 2014
Reprint: 2015

Published by Satish Kumar Jain for
CBS Publishers & Distributors Pvt Ltd
4819/XI Prahlad Street, 24 Ansari Road, Daryaganj, New Delhi 110 002, India.
Ph: 23289259, 23266861, 23266867   Website: www.cbspd.com
Fax: 011-23243014   e-mail: delhi@cbspd.com; cbspubs@airtelmail.in.
Corporate Office: 204 FIE, Industrial Area, Patparganj, Delhi 110 092
Ph: 4934 4934   Fax: 4934 4935   e-mail: publishing@cbspd.com; publicity@cbspd.com

Branches

- **Bengaluru:** Seema House 2975, 17th Cross, K.R. Road,
  Banasankari 2nd Stage, Bengaluru 560 070, Karnataka
  Ph: +91-80-26771678/79   Fax: +91-80-26771680   e-mail: bangalore@cbspd.com
- **Chennai:** 20, West Park Road, Shenoy Nagar, Chennai 600 030, Tamil Nadu
  Ph: +91-44-26260666, 26208620   Fax: +91-44-42032115   e-mail: chennai@cbspd.com
- **Kochi:** 36/14 Kalluvilakam, Lissie Hospital Road, Kochi 682 018, Kerala
  Ph: +91-484-4059061-65   Fax: +91-484-4059065   e-mail: kochi@cbspd.com
- **Mumbai:** 83-C, Dr E Moses Road, Worli, Mumbai-400018, Maharashtra
  Ph: +91-22-24902340/41   Fax: +91-22-24902342   e-mail: mumbai@cbspd.com
- **Pune:** Bhuruk Prestige, Sr. No. 52/12/2+1+3/2 Narhe, Haveli
  (Near Katraj-Dehu Road Bypass), Pune 411 041, Maharashtra
  Ph: +91-20-64704058/59, 32392277   Fax: +91-20-24300160   e-mail: pune@cbspd.com

Representatives

- **Hyderabad**   0-9885175004
- **Nagpur**   0-9021734563
- **Vijayawada**   0-9000660880
- **Kolkata**   0-9831437309, 0-9051152362
- **Patna**   0-9334159340

Printed at Manipal Technologies Limited

to
our amazing grandson who suffered
hypoglycemia resulting in brain injury
at AIIMS, New Delhi,
due to hard fixed beliefs and practices,
and the consequent negligence of newborn care experts.
He has learnt to fight all odds, despite the permanent
disability including cerebral palsy and visual impairment
(see hypoglycemia on page 90)

Preface

India continues to have rampant maternal undernutrition/ anemia, responsible for high maternal deaths, and a large number of low birth weight deliveries (28–30%). These low birth weight infants continue as undernourished children and increase to 42% by 3 years of age. They suffer from poor growth and development of brain in the later weeks of pregnancy to 20th months of life due to maternal undernutrition and faulty weaning practices. The government programmes and other services have made a little dent in this cycle of undernutrition and infection (National Family Health Surveys II and III).

We have made scientific attempt to prepare this guide for "maternal child care givers" and the family to understand the Principles of Child Care: Conception to Childhood.

KN Agarwal
DK Agarwal

Acknowledgements

We are thankful to Shri Dharmesh Agarwal, Creative Designer, Textile Studio, B-48, Hosiery Complex, Noida Phase II (UP), for designing the cover and shooting the children in action. Our thanks are also due to Mrs Sabitha S S, Sister incharge Neonatal Care Unit, Metro General Hospital, Noida (UP), for taking pictures of the newborn.

Contents

Contents

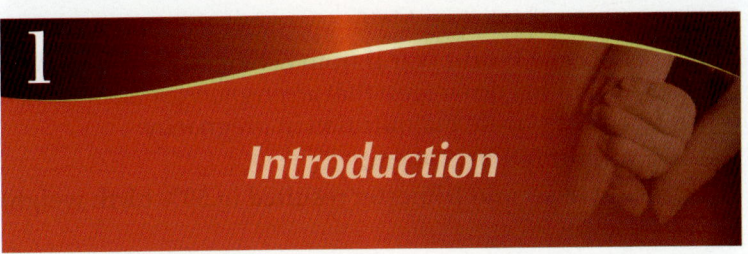

1

Introduction

A. YOUR NUTRITION IN PREGNANCY

The evidences that *nutrition in pregnancy* is important are discussed in (a) births from rural undernourished women, and (b) experiences of world war II, showing that *prepregnancy nutrition* (in Russia *vs* Holland) did affect birth weight differently.

The importance of special nutrients like *folic acid* and iron (anemia) is also discussed. Finally, the dietary requirement to form "balanced diet in pregnancy and lactation" are presented.

Pregnancy (*Understand Importance of Nutrition*)

A. Why Nutrition is Important for Baby and You?

Rural pregnancy data from Varanasi (1987–1993), Indian Pediatrics 2000 and 2002 showed that:

- 27.4% babies at birth were small in size (< 2500 gm),
- 6.6% were preterm births (born before full term), and
- Only 8.2% weighed > 3000 gm (normal birth weight being around 3.3 kg).

More births with weight < 2500 gm, were due to **maternal undernutrition** resulting in fetal growth arrest. These women in later pregnancy (during 35–43 weeks of gestation) showed weekly weight gain of 15–25 gm, only. In contrast, women in Ludhiana gained > 100 gm per week. This was due to poor nutrition in prepregnancy and pregnancy period.

Nutrition supplementation and correction of anemia in pregnancy improves birth weight and maternal weight. Let us discuss the importance of prepregnancy nutrition.

1

B. Prepregnancy Nutrition Matters

The experience of **World War II** from Leningrad(USSR) famine (period 16 months) do suggest that *prepregnancy undernutrition* when faced with acute malnutrition in pregnancy:

- **Birth weight fell by 530 gm;**
- **Exposure in second trimester resulted in 50% birth weight < 2500 gm.**

In contrast, Dutch famine was imposed on a *previously well-nourished population.* It reduced birth weight by 327 gm and corresponding figure for those with weight < 2500 gm was 9% only.

These studies convince us that prepregnancy nutrition is important for health of child and mother.

For mothers, it is important to learn that **nutrition prior to conception, during pregnancy, and in lactation** makes foundation of a **healthy child**.

It is established now that baby listens in womb in last trimester (last weeks of pregnancy)—see TIMES Magazine July 2013.

C. Importance of Special Nutrients in Pregnancy

1. **Folic acid supplementation** during the periconceptional period (about one month before and one month after conception) dramatically reduces the incidence of devastating birth defects of brain and spinal cord called **neural tube defects,** i.e. **anencephaly** or **spina bifida.**

2. Periconceptional **multivitamin** supplementation **with folic acid** may protect against congenital heart malformations.

Thus, folic acid supplementation (at least 400–800 mcg/day) is recommended for all women capable of becoming pregnant. Women who have had a previous *neural tube defects* (brain or spinal cord defect) or any other congenital malformation, affected pregnancy may be advised to consume up to 4 mg/day (4,000 mcg/day) of folic acid if they are planning a pregnancy.

There were significant beneficiary effects of maternal intake of folic acid along with multivitamins and iron in early pregnancy, as there was reduced:

a. Incidence of brain tumors (primitive neuroectodermal tumors)

b. Daily intake of vitamins and minerals one month before and in pregnancy reduced neuroblastoma by 30–40% in children

c. Periconceptional use of vitamins in Down syndrome reduced risk of acute lymphoblastic leukemia by 63%.

So there are significant advantages of eating folic acid, multi-vitamins and iron in prepregnancy and during early months of pregnancy.

> Why pregnancy nutrition is important
>
> Brain growth, development of neurotransmitters maximum from 20th week of fetal life
>
> Baby listens in the last trimester
> TIMES Magazine July 2013

Pregnancy anemia—means pregnant or lactating women have lower hemoglobin than normal. In pregnancy, hemoglobin physiologically lowers due to hem dilution.

a. Prevalence in India

- Indian Council of Medical Research 2001 showed that 84.7% mothers are anemic (hemoglobin < 11.0 gm%). Of these, 9.9% are with severe anemia(hemoglobin < 7.0 gm%).
- Agarwal et al (Indian J Med Res 2006) showed in 7 states that pregnancy anemia was in 86.1% women (severe anemia in 9.7%); anemia during lactation being 81.7% (severe anemia 7%). Thus, pregnancy/lactation anemia is a serious health hazard for mother and child in India.

b. Health Consequences of Anemia in Pregnancy

1. It has been clearly demonstrated that the anemic **pregnant woman is at greater risk of death** during the prenatal period. Close to 500,000 mothers die in childbirth or early post-partum period every year, the vast majority taking place in the developing world. **Anemia is the major contributory or sole cause in 20–40% of maternal deaths.** In 2012, India recorded more maternal deaths than any other country in the world (around 56,000 per year). One maternal death was recorded every 10 minutes in India (2013).

2. Anemic pregnant women had a higher **risk of preterm delivery** in relation to nonanemic women.

3. The more severe the anemia, the greater the **risk of low birth weight** (baby weighs less than expected for the gestational age).

4. Fetal iron stores are reduced in iron deficiency—result in **poor fetal brain neurotransmitter** development. Such brain changes cannot be corrected on later life treatment.

5. Baby has low iron stores so develops **anemia in early infancy.**

6. Anemic mothers have poor work capacity.

c. Iron Needs of Pregnancy

Iron needs exhibit a marked increase during the second and especially during the third trimester when median daily needs increase up to an average of 5.6 mg per day (that is, 4.1 mg above median prepregnancy needs). The requirement is ≈0.8 mg Fe in the first trimester, between 4 and 5 mg in the second trimester, and > 6 mg in the third trimester. Much of this will be available from the balanced diet. However, folate + iron tablet with 500–600 µg folate + 30 mg iron as supplement will work.

Factor	Milligrams of iron	
	Range	Median
Fetal iron	200–450	270
Placental iron	30–170	80
Partum and puerperium losses	90–310	250
Hemoglobin and tissue expansion	130–430	200
Maintenance during amenorrhea	160–220	190
Subtotal 1 (total iron costs)	610–1580	990
Postpartum involution iron	130–430	200
Total	480–1150	790

B. BALANCED DIET IN PREGNANCY AND LACTATION

Basically "balanced diet in pregnancy" must contain things from the entire food groups. It should be proper in quantity and quality.

A. Nutritional Needs in Pregnancy

Prepregnancy Diet

The diet during, even before, pregnancy has to be rich in calories, proteins, vitamins and minerals and balanced.

Pregnancy Diet

Your pregnancy brings in physiological and emotional changes as well as poses extra demands on the body. For a successful pregnancy, body needs extra nutrition:

- For the developing fetus,
- Pregnant woman herself, and
- For the lactation period to follow.

These nutritional demands have to be met for a healthy child and mother.

The most essential period when you have to take care of your 'Pregnancy Diet' is during the first three months when the principal organs both external and internal and the nervous system of the baby are formed. So begin a nourishing diet right from start even if you face discomfort like nausea. This is important if you want your baby to have an optimal growth.

A well-balanced nutritious diet consists of proteins, fats, carbohydrates, minerals and vitamins all in one plate. You essentially need to have a 'Pregnancy Diet' comprised of a variety of foods selected from the five food groups (Fig. 1.1–modified for Indians).

1. Fats and sweets (use small amount)
2. Milk, yogurt, and cheese group (4 servings)
3. Meat, poultry, fish, dry beans, eggs, and nuts group (3 servings, 5 servings for teen pregnancy)
4. Vegetable group fruit group (3–5 servings)
5. Bread, cereal, rice and dosa, idli, dhokla group (6–11 servings)

These five FOOD groups in daily diet will get you all the nutrients you need. Apart from the natural supplements, folic acid, iron, and calcium are of utmost importance and are often prescribed by the obstetricians.

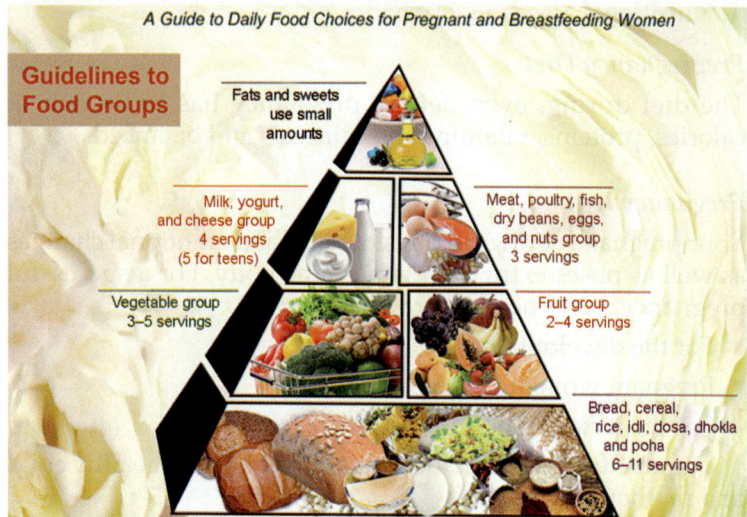

Fig. 1.1: Food guide pyramid

Have a variety of food each day and avoid sticking to the same kind of food. However, try variations in moderation. Be sure to listen to your body when you consider the amount of food you need to take. Your appetite is the best guide. Normally try and have at least three proper meals a day. You can also break it into six smaller meals in case you have problems like nausea or heartburns.

The needs vary in the three trimesters. Generally, the gestation period in humans is 40 weeks.

Energy: The energy needs of the body increase by 300 kcal per day in 2nd and 3rd trimesters.

Pregnancy = 2600 kcal; Lactation= 2700 kcal

Calories are needed to cater the growing demands of the fetus and the mother, and to accumulate fat stores which act as reserves during lactation. Considerable weight gain about 10–14 kg during pregnancy is desirable.

Proteins: An additional 15 gm/day of protein has to be supplied in the diet. Complete and good quality proteins in the form of milk, legumes, pulses, nuts, whole grains, meat, egg and cheese will help.

Protein = 65 gm during pregnancy and lactation

Fats: In healthy mothers, the fetal organs already have stores of fat and so additional fat is not required. Nevertheless, essential fatty acids (EFA) should be supplied during pregnancy. Some of the food sources of omega-3 and omega-6 fatty acids are *fish* and *shellfish, flaxseed (linseed), soya oil, canola (rapeseed) oil, chia seeds, pumpkin seeds, sunflower seeds, leafy vegetables,* and *walnuts.*

Two polyunsaturated fatty acids (PUFAs) that cannot be made in the body are linoleic acid and alpha-linolenic acid. These must be provided by diet and are known as essential fatty acids. Within the body, both can be converted to other PUFAs such as arachidonic acid, or eicosapentaenoic acid (EPA) and docosahexaenoic acid (DHA).

In the body, PUFAs are important for i) maintaining the membranes of all cells and ii) making prostaglandins which regulate many body processes which include inflammation and blood clotting.

Another requirement for fat in the diet is to enable the fat-soluble vitamins A, D, E and K to be absorbed from food; and for regulating body cholesterol metabolism.

Polyunsaturated Fatty Acids—Dietary Sources

Food sources of the two main dietary polyunsaturated fatty acids (linoleic acid and alpha-linolenic acid) are listed below.

Linoleic Acid (Omega-6 Family)

- Vegetables
- Fruits
- Nuts
- Grains
- Seeds

Good Sources

Oils made from:
- Safflower
- Sunflower
- Corn
- Soya
- Evening primrose
- Pumpkin
- Wheat germ

Alpha-Linolenic Acid (Omega-3 Family)

(Please note – fish is not the only source of omega-3 acids.).

- Flaxseeds(linseeds)
- Mustard seeds
- Hemp seeds
- Walnut oil(walnuts)
- Green leafy vegetables
- Grains
- Spirulina

Good Sources

Oils made from:

- Linseed(flaxseeds)
- Rapeseed(canola)

Research shows that adequate levels of omega-3 fatty acids enhance

- development of the fetal and infant brain and may improve cognitive development,
- visual acuity, hand-eye coordination and attention span,
- that maternal omega-3 fatty acid intake lowers the infant's risk of developing allergies and asthma later in life,
- also very important for maternal well-being. Not only do they protect from cardiovascular disease, lower triglyceride levels but also may prevent inflammatory diseases like rheumatoid arthritis. They also have a specific effect on maternal health and the outcome of pregnancy, and
- appear to reduce incidence of pre-eclampsia, preterm labor and the risk for prenatal and postpartum depression.

You can eat fish oil capsules as medicine. This will be good for you and baby's brain.

Micronutrients during Pregnancy

Vitamins: Folic acid 600 µg, biotin 30 µg, niacin 18 mg, pantothenic acid 6 mg, riboflavin 1.4 mg, A–2500 IU, B_6–1.9 mg, B_{12}–2.6 µg, C–80 mg, D–600 IU, E–15 mg, K–75 µg.

Minerals: Calcium 1300 mg (200–250 mg daily of calcium is transferred to fetus in the 3rd trimester), magnesium 400 mg, phosphorus 1250 mg, iodine 220 µg, iron 27 mg, magnesium 400 µg, potassium 4700 mg, sodium 1500 mg, zinc 12 µg, copper 1 mg/day.

Micronutrients (vitamins+minerals) are available in green vegetables/fruits in balanced diet (Fig. 1.2). Commercial tablets provide needed micronutrients. Needed calcium is available in 4 cups of milk (around 300 mg in a cup). For iron and folic acid, we have tablets supplied at all government health centers and are commercially available.

Principles of Good Balanced Diet

1. No dieting, avoid stress, be happy.
2. Plenty of fruits (citrus) and vegetables—green and colored.
3. Small regular frequent feeds.
4. Whole/multigrain cereals, dairy foods (milk, curd, cheese)
5. Iron rich foods (boil milk and cook vegetables in cast iron utensils).
6. Limit fried foods/salt/spices.
7. Protein—dairy products, legumes, egg, fish, and lean meat.
8. Some fat/oil/fish oil.
9. 6–7 glasses filtered water.
10. Limit tea, coffee as caffeine can affect baby's sleep.

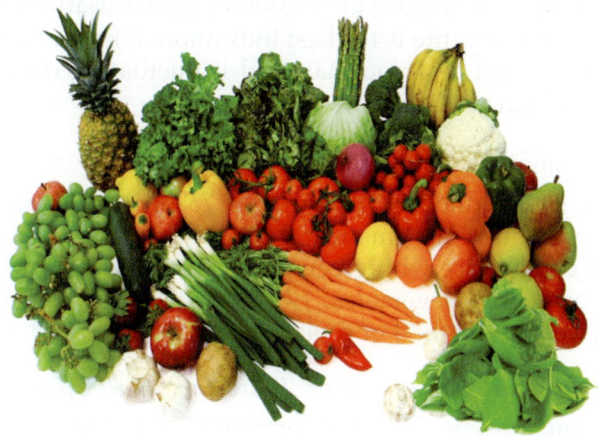

Fig. 1.2: Vegetables and fruits provide vitamins/minerals/antioxidants

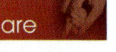
Eat a variety of foods from these different food groups each day:

- *Milk and dairy products:* Skimmed milk, yogurt, buttermilk, paneer. These foods are high in calcium, protein and vitamin B_{12}.

- *Cereals, whole grains, pulses and nuts:* These are good sources of proteins for vegetarians. Vegetarians need about 45 gm of nuts and 2/3 of a cup of legumes for protein each day. One egg, 14 gm of nuts, or 1/4 cup of legumes is considered equivalent to roughly 28 gm of meat, poultry, or fish.

- *Vegetables and fruits:* These provide vitamins, minerals and fiber.

- *Meat, fish and poultry:* These provide concentrated proteins.

- *Fluids:* Drink lots of fluids, especially water and fresh fruit juices. Make sure you drink clean filtered water. Carry your own water when out of the house, or buy bottled water from a reputed brand. *Most diseases are caused by waterborne bacteria/viruses.* Go easy on packaged juices as they have very high sugar content.

- *Fats and oils:* Ghee, butter, coconut milk, and oil are high in saturated fats, which are not very healthy. Hydrogenated (vanaspati and dalda) oils are high in trans fats, which are as bad for you as saturated fats. A better source of fat is vegetable oils because these contain more unsaturated fat.

Your own appetite is the best indication of how much food you need to eat and you may find it fluctuating during the course of your pregnancy.

B. Recommended Nutrient Intake

Pregnancy: Around 2600 kcal; protein 75 gm. Diet should have 3–4 cups of milk; 100 gm meat/fish; 3–4 eggs per week (vegetarians can replace with green gram, cottage cheese, yogurt); green or yellow vegetables; 1/2 cup citrus and other fruits (2 services); chapatis–4 or replace with rice.

Mixed Diet with Good Flavor, Taste and Small Sweet Dish

Lactation: Around 2700 kcal; protein 65 g and rest pattern is similar to pregnancy.

Diet is divided in 6 meals—**breakfast, mid morning meal, lunch, mid afternoon meal, tea and dinner.**

C. What to Limit in Diet?

- Avoid known allergic food to mother. Following tips will help you and your baby stay healthy.

- **Intake of vitamin A must be controlled** because it may cause damage to embryo. However, pro-vitamin A from green vegetables, carrots, etc. are safe in pregnancy.

- Cabbage, cauliflower and all long green vegetables such as turai, louki, parwal, spinach, govari should be used alternately. You must keep a balance, rather than eating same vegetable all the time.

- Those who suffer from constipation, gas, bloating must avoid peas and other 'heavy to digest' cereals, potato. They may take green gram as it is easy to digest and gives protein.

- Black grapes, banana, ripe mango, dates, cashew nuts, apricot are very beneficial.

- Butter, clarified butter, milk, honey, fennel seeds, sweets made from jaggery rather than white sugar can be taken in small quantity.

- Rice, murmure, pulao, bhakari, khichdi, chapati, paratha, Gujarati thepla are the items made from wheat and rice, so they are quite beneficial. Idli made of dal and rice is a good food.

- Items such as sandwich, bakery bread, bun, dhokla, pizza, khandva, pancake, khaman, steamed rice cake, curd, tomato, tamarind, kadhi usually increase the swelling and acidity. So, try to avoid such items, but if such problems do not exist, you can take in small quantity.

Indian women try to carry out fasts during pregnancy which is not good for "fetal" health.

- Reduce brinjal, suran/yam, papaya, celery, onion, chilli, garlic, ginger, pepper, asafetida, mustard, bajara, carom seeds, jaggery from your diet. You must remember that those who have previous history of abortion better they must avoid these.

- Do not eat left over, frozen and deep-frozen food.

- Avoid cold drinks, mutton, cocoa, chicken, eggs, alcohol, smoking, tobacco, betel nut, pan-masala, but tea, coffee and ice-creams can be taken in small quantity.
- Remember, the baby inside depends on you for proper nutrition. So, if you will take healthy and balanced diet your child will become healthy.
- During pregnancy, mother must focus on supplemental nutrients while maintaining a balanced and nutritious diet. They must get a list of healthy Indian foods and meal planning tips from doctor to eat well during pregnancy.

Indian women must maintain a high quality diet during their pregnancy to get a healthy, fit and fine baby. Now start following your diet chart to become a healthy mother (Table 1.1).

The best rule is to eat when you are hungry and to choose healthy food rather than calorie-rich dishes with little nutritive value.

Table 1.1: Healthy diet menu—flexible can be modified, eat different things to cover all groups of nutrients

Option	Early morning	Breakfast	Mid morning	Lunch	Evening	Dinner
1.	Mixed dry fruits-milkshake	Whole wheat or mixed grain roti or toast, or dhokla or vegetable omeleltte, walnuts/cashew nuts	Creamy spinach soup	Paratha (low oil), vegetable-carrot peas, kofta curry raitha, sprouted beans salad	Mixed vegetable small uttappam or idli, apple	Brown rice, dal fry, palak paneer, green salad
2.	Pasteurized milk	Vegetable patties or fruit salad, and spinach paratha with yoghurt or butter, apricot	Tomato soup	Plain roti, toor dal, cauliflower, rice and vegetable salad, kheer(low sugar)	Cheese-tomato/cucumber sandwich or fruity smoothie banana and strawberry, peanut cookies	Vegetable biriyani, apple salad, yogurt (fat free)

(contd.)

Table 1.1: Healthy diet menu—flexible can be modified, eat different things to cover all groups of nutrients (*Contd.*)

Option	Early morning	Breakfast	Mid morning	Lunch	Evening	Dinner
3.	Pure apple juice	Poha or oats porridge or cheese sandwich or mixed bean cutlet, dates	Vegetables + tomato + basil soup	Paneer stuffed/ dosai/or paratha, dal fry, raita and jeera rice	Fresh hot carrot or lauki halwa [sweet]	Moong dal khichdi, veg. curry and paratha
4.	Almond milk	Veg cutlets or wheat rava upma with veggies, orange juice, dried sweet fig [anjeer]	Mixed vegetable soup	Lemon peas rice, cabbage and moong dal, mint raitha, small mango/ fruit	Bread cutlet or gobi matter samosa, apricot and an apple juice	Plain rotis of whole wheat with alu methi sabji, buttermilk
5.	Tomato and/or carrot juice	Plain rotis of whole wheat with alu methi sabji, butter milk	Vegetable soup	Vegetable khichdi, roti or bhakari, peas curry, black grapes	Lemon sevai, dried dates, dried fruits, a green tea	Vegetable pulao, buttermilk, bhakari or plain paratha

D. Problems in Pregnancy and Dietary Suggestions

- In the first few weeks of pregnancy, you may not feel like eating proper meals, especially if you suffer from morning sickness, nausea. Try then to eat smaller but more frequent meals throughout the day.

The initial months are the most difficult for pregnant women. It is common for them to suffer from morning sickness, diarrhea, and/or constipation. It gets especially difficult to hold food down without vomiting it out. Following are some dietary suggestions for pregnant women in India to overcome this difficult phase:

- **Morning sickness** can be tackled by eating light (low salt puffed rice with Bengal gram) biscuits or cereal before you even get out of bed. Opt for small, but frequent meals, spread throughout the day. Avoid food that is fried, rich in fats, and greasy because it only further worsen the discomfort.

- **Constipation** can be dealt with by consuming fresh fruits and vegetables. Drinking 6–8 glasses of water a day is also known to be of great help.

- To deal with **diarrhea,** women would need to eat more food that contain pectin and gums, which are two essential types of dietary fiber that help to absorb excess water in the body. Examples of such foods include bananas, white rice and oatmeal.

- You can deal with **heartburn** by eating small and frequent meals spread throughout the day. Try drinking a glass of milk before sitting down to eat. Also limit your intake of caffeinated foods and beverages.

C. WEIGHT GAIN IN PREGNANCY

Most women gain between 10 and 15 kg, but too much weight gain should be avoided. However, the weight gain during pregnancy will vary according to your prepregnancy weight. According to the experts, an overweight woman is advised to gain only 7 kg and an underweight woman to gain up to 18 kg (Tables 1.2 and 1.3).

For this, limit on too much fat and sugar in your diet.

Table 1.2: Weight gain for ideal pregnant women (there are individual variations)

Your prepregnancy height (m=meter) and weight (kg) as rough guide

Height	Underweight	Normal	Overweight	Obese
1.52 m	< 46	46.0–60.0	60–66.5	> 67
1.57 m	< 48.5	48.5–63.5	63.8–71	> 72
1.63 m	< 52.5	52.5–68.8	69.0–77.0	> 77.5
1.68 m	< 55.5	55.6–72.8	73–81.5	> 82
1.78 m	< 62.5	62.5–82.0	82–91.5	> 92
Your gain plan (kg)				
if you were…	underweight	normal	overweight	obese
Reasonable weight gain in kg	13–18	11–16	8–12	< 8

Table 1.3: Alterations in body composition during pregnancy. How the pregnancy weight gain of 11–12 kg is distributed?

Maternal stores of nutrients and muscle development	3 kg
Increased body fluid	2 kg
Increased blood	1.5–2 kg
Breast growth	600 gm
Enlarged uterus	1 kg
Amniotic fluid	1 kg
Placenta	600 gm
Baby	3.4–4 kg
Total	11–16 kg

On a Trimester Basis

- **First trimester:** Most women put on around 1.6 kg in the first three months.

- **Second trimester:** Around 0.5 kg a week for the next three months (5.5–6.4 kg) in total.

- **Third trimester:** Only around 5 kg over the last three months.

Do Not Eat For Two: Many pregnant women wrongly think that they should eat for two. Note that **you need only 200–300 extra calories daily in pregnancy,** i.e. a cup of reduced fat milk or yogurt and a medium orange. This is because **your body actually absorbs more nutrients from food you eat during pregnancy.**

The goal of pregnancy is to have a healthy baby. Maintaining healthy and steady weight gain during pregnancy promotes overall health and reduces the incidence of prenatal morbidity and mortality. This, in turn, has a positive effect on the baby's general health and brain development.

Since conditions during pregnancy will have long-term effects on adult health, "moderation" should be taken into account for both dietary and physical activity recommendations. Most importantly, the total recommended pregnancy weight gain depends on prepregnant body weight, and weight issues should be addressed before pregnancy (Table 1.2).

Key Notes

- In our country, maternal undernutrition and anemia are rampant affecting fetal growth and brain growth, increase low birth weight deliveries associated with later life diabetes, hypertension, and coronary heart diseases.
- Balanced diet (macro and micronutrients) as per food pyramid be taken even before pregnancy.
- Folic acid, calcium and iron are needed in higher quantities during pregnancy and lactation.
- Folic acid alone at least 1 month before conception and in first trimester prevents "neural defects" and in association with other micronutrients reduces some cancers.
- Mothers with low weight should gain more weight to achieve good pregnancy outcome and for lactation (12–18 kg)—obese mothers should gain less weight (7 kg).

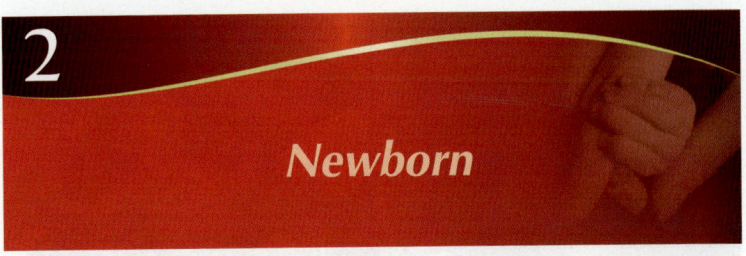

2

Newborn

A. NEWBORN AT BIRTH

In this chapter, newborn at birth (term and preterm) and care of cord are discussed.

A **newborn** is an infant who is only hours, days, or up to a few weeks old. In medical contexts, newborn or **neonate** refers to an infant in the first 28 days after birth.

Full term (FT) infants: Gestation—37 to < 42 weeks.

Premature (born before complete pregnancy period) infants: Born before completion of 37 weeks.

Post mature (born after the full term of the pregnancy) infants: Delivered after 42 weeks of gestation.

Before birth: The term fetus is used.

Newborn Babies Seconds after Birth (Fig. 2.1)

Typically, a full term newborn baby has the following characteristic appearance:

- *Weight:* Average 3.4 kg (range 2.7–4.6 kg). Babies below 2.5 kg at birth are considered to be low birth weight and need special evaluation.

- *Length:* Approximately 50 cm. Remember, small women have small babies and many genetic factors also play a role in determining the length of the baby.

- *Head:* Your baby's head appears large for the body and may have an elongated shape or appear to have some 'bumps'. This is due to changes called molding, which occurs in labour and delivery. Small bumps called 'caput' usually disappear in 1–2 days. Soon the head gets rounder. The head circumference is 33–35 cm.

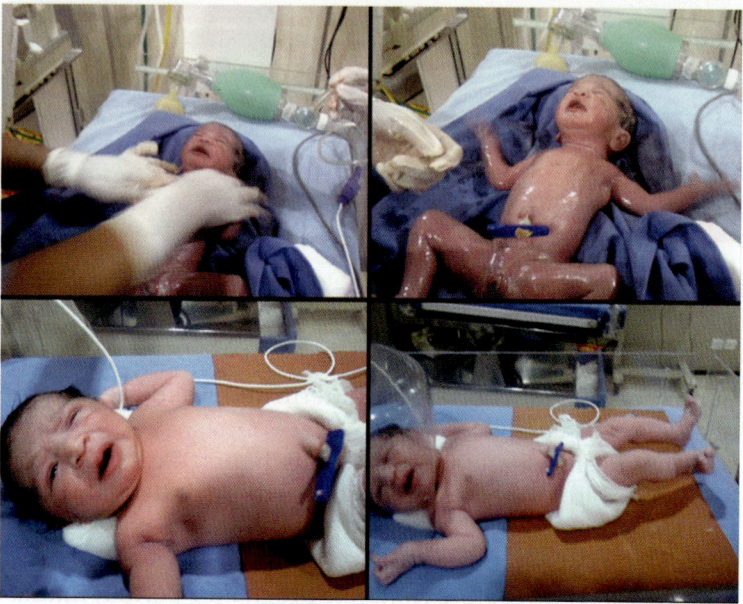

Fig. 2.1: Cleaning the baby after birth and giving oxygen

- *Soft spots or fontanelles:* There are 2 areas on the head, where bone formation is incomplete at birth. The larger one, in front of the head closes by 6–18 months. The smaller one at the back usually closes by 6 weeks.

- *Hair:* As all people vary, so does their hair. Your baby may have lots of hair or none at all! It depends on familial and racial factors.

- *Heart beats:* Usually the heart rate is 120–140 beats per minute.

- *Respiratory rate (breathing):* It is faster than adults, usually 30–40 breaths/minute. Breathing may be noisy or stop for many seconds. This is not uncommon.

- *Colour:* Depending on the parents, the skin colour of newborn varies. In general, newborn babies look flushed and pink all over. However, the palms and soles of the feet may look dusky or little bluish.

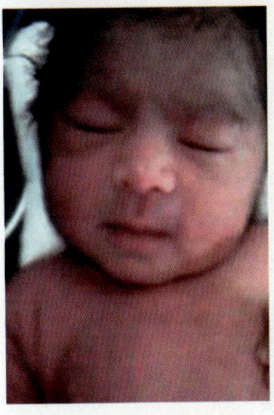

Fig. 2.2: Newborn after 2–3 hours

Newborn (Fig. 2.2)

- Most of the newborn babies are born vigorous-strong respiratory efforts, good muscle tone, heart rate >100/min.
- 10% need assistance
- 1% major resuscitation measure to survive
- Was the baby born FT?
- Is amniotic fluid clear of meconeum and no evidence of infection?
- Baby breathing and crying?
- Has good muscle tone?

Body length: The average range for length of newborns is 46–50 cm, although premature newborns may be much smaller (short).

Birth weight: The average weight of a full term newborn is approximately 3.4 kg (and is typically in the range of 2.7–4.6 kg). Over the first 5–7 days following birth, the body weight of a term neonate decreases by 3–7%, and is largely a result of the resorption and urination of the fluid that initially fills the lungs, in addition to a delay of often a few days before breastfeeding becomes effective. After the first week, healthy term neonates should gain 10–20 gm/kg/day.

Head circumference: During labour/birth, the infant's skull changes shape to fit through the birth canal, sometimes causing the child to be born with a misshapen or elongated head. It usually returns to normal on its own within a few days or weeks.

Circumference for a full term infant is 33–36 cm at birth. At birth, many regions of the newborn's skull have not yet been converted to bone, leaving "soft spots" known as fontanels. The two largest are the diamond-shaped **anterior (frontal) fontanel,** located at the top front portion of the head, and the smaller triangular-shaped **posterior (occipital) fontanel,** which lies at the back of the head. Later in the child's life, these bones will fuse together in a natural process (Fig. 2.3).

Frontal fontanel

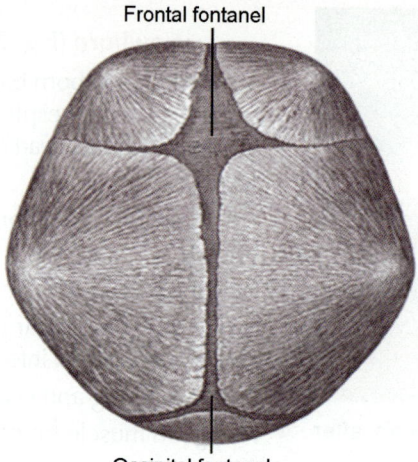

Occipital fontanel

Fig. 2.3: Frontal and occipital fontanels

Preterm Baby (Figs 2.4 and 2.5)

Premature babies have a number of characteristics depending on their gestational age.

- *Skin:* May be reddened. The skin may be thin so blood vessels are easily seen.

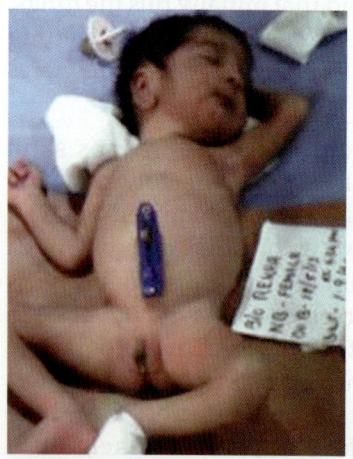

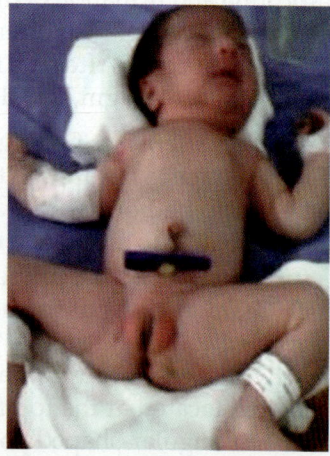

Fig. 2.4: Preterm wt: 1.9 kg; gestation: 33 wk; age: 8 days

Fig. 2.5: Preterm 35 wk wt: 2.2 kg

- *Lanugo:* There is a lot of fine hair all over the baby's body.

- *Limbs:* The limbs are thin and may be poorly flexed or floppy due to poor muscle tone.

- *Head size:* Appears large in proportion to the body. The **fontanelles** (open spaces where skull bones join) are smooth and flat.

- *Chest:* No breast tissue before 34 weeks of pregnancy.

- *Sucking ability:* Weak or absent.

- *Genitals:* In boys, the testes may not be descended and the scrotum may be small; in girls, the clitoris and labia minora may be large.

- *Soles of feet:* Creases are located only in the anterior (front) of the sole, not all over as in the term baby.

The physical growth pattern in children and the growth curves are given at the end (*see* p 67–74).

B. UMBILICAL CORD

During pregnancy, the umbilical cord supplies nutrients and oxygen to your developing baby. After birth, the umbilical cord is no longer needed—so it is clamped and snipped. This leaves behind a short stump. The umbilical cord does not contain pain-sensitive nerve fibers, so your baby would not feel any discomfort.

How to care for your newborn's umbilical cord stump? Until the stump dries out and falls off, keep it clean and dry. Usually in 7 to 21 days, the stump will dry up and drop off; leaving a small wound that may take a few days to heal.

A newborn's umbilical cord stump typically falls off within about two weeks after birth. In the meantime, treat your baby's umbilical cord stump gently (Fig. 2.6).

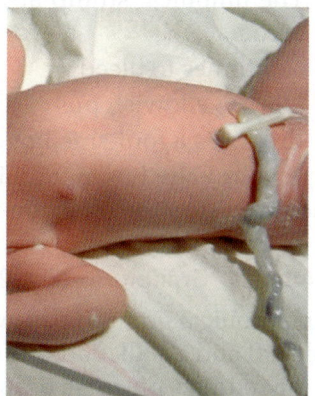

Fig. 2.6: Umbilical cord of 3–4 min old newborn

Taking Care of the Stump

Your baby's umbilical cord stump will change from *yellowish green* to *brown* to *black* as it dries out and eventually falls off— usually within about two weeks after birth. In the meantime, treat the area gently.

- *Keep the stump clean:* In routine, the diaper should not cover the stump. If the stump becomes dirty or sticky, then clean it with filtered water and dry it by holding a clean, absorbent cloth around the stump or fanning it with a piece of paper.

- *Keep the stump dry:* Expose the stump to air to help dry out the base. Keep the front of your baby's diaper folded down to avoid covering the stump. In warm weather, dress your baby in a diaper and T-shirt to improve air circulation.

- *Stick with sponge baths:* Sponge baths might be most practical during the healing process. When the stump falls off, you can bathe your baby in a baby tub or sink.

- *Let the stump fall off:* DO NOT pull off the stump yourself, even if it is hanging on by only a thread.

Signs of Umbilical Cord Infection

During the cord stump healing process, it is normal to see a little crust or dried blood near the stump.
- The umbilical stump appears red and swollen around the cord
- Continues to bleed
- Oozes yellowish pus
- Produces a foul-smelling discharge

If your baby has an umbilical cord infection, prompt treatment can stop the infection from spreading.

Umbilical Granuloma (Fig. 2.7)

An umbilical granuloma is when the baby's cord dries up and falls off and a stalk of tissue still remains. It looks like a pink to light reddish piece of tissue. The granuloma will not grow normal skin tissue on top of it, and will ooze mucous until it is treated.

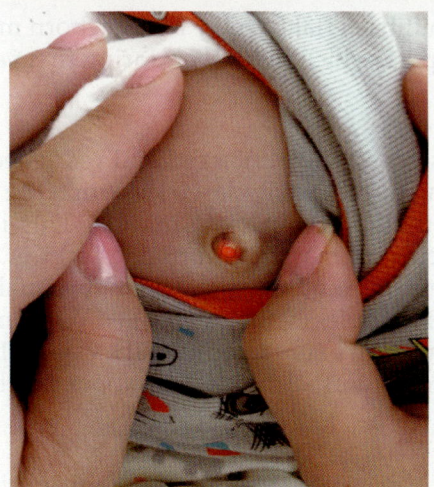

Fig. 2.7: Umbilical granuloma in a newborn

Treatment: The first line of treatment is usually

a. The **salt crystal** dip in water, then apply on the granuloma

or

b. The chemical **silver nitrate,** take a stick of the chemical and carefully apply it to the granuloma to dry it up.

This process may take several treatments before the granuloma is finally gone.

Hair

Some newborns have a fine, downy body hair called lanugo. It may be particularly noticeable on the back, shoulders, forehead, ears and face of premature infants. Lanugo disappears within a few weeks.

Infants may be born with full heads of hair; others may have very fine hair or may even be bald.

Skin

Immediately after birth, a newborn's skin is often grayish to dusky blue in color. As soon as the newborn begins to breathe, usually within a minute or two, the skin's color reaches its normal tone. Newborns are wet, covered in streaks of blood, and coated with a white substance known as vernix caseosa,

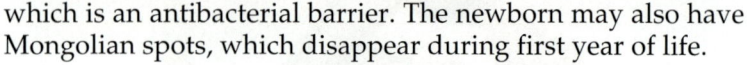
which is an antibacterial barrier. The newborn may also have Mongolian spots, which disappear during first year of life.

Genitals

A newborn's genitals are enlarged and reddened, with male infants having an unusually large scrotum. The breasts may also be enlarged, even in male infants. This is caused by naturally occurring maternal hormones and is a temporary condition. Females (and even males) may actually discharge milk from their nipples (sometimes called Witch milk), and/or a bloody or milky-like substance from the vagina. In either case, this is considered normal and will disappear with time.

Key Notes

- 10% of all babies need assistance to initiate "first breathe", so a trained health care giver along with a pediatrician should attend your delivery.
- Preterm babies may require special respiratory assistance and should be delivered in a hospital with "newborn care unit".
- Umbilical cord needs care, do not cover it, learn signs of infection and consult your pediatrician for any suspicion.

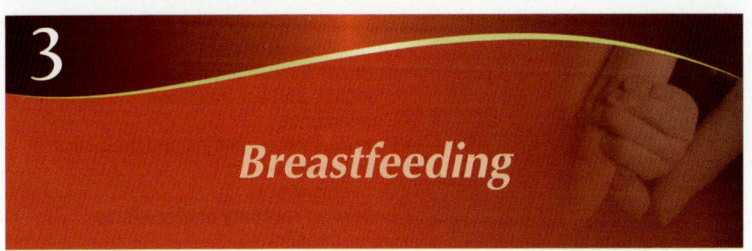

3

Breastfeeding

Breast care, correction for flat or inverted nipples, diet during breastfeeding and burping are discussed.

A. LACTATION

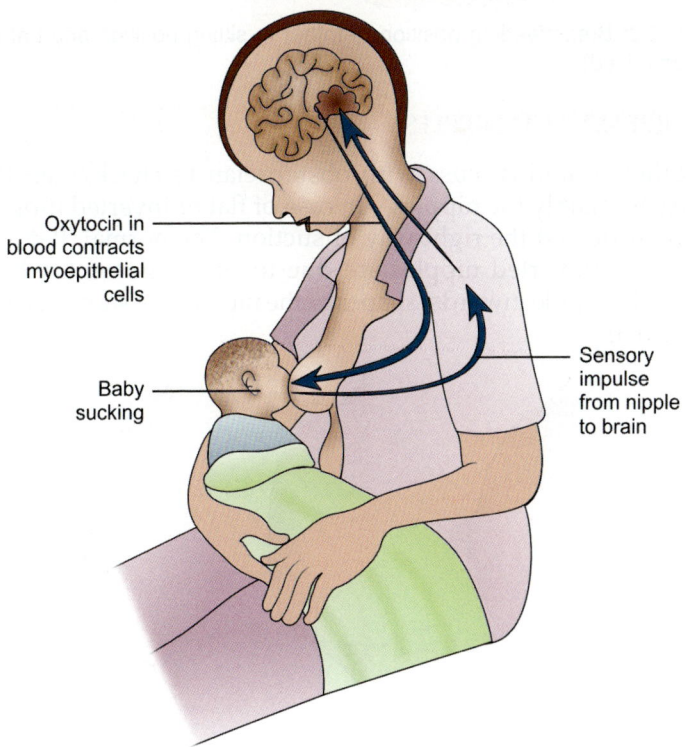

Oxytocin in blood contracts myoepithelial cells

Baby sucking

Sensory impulse from nipple to brain

Fig. 3.1: Brain control through hormones on breast milk flow

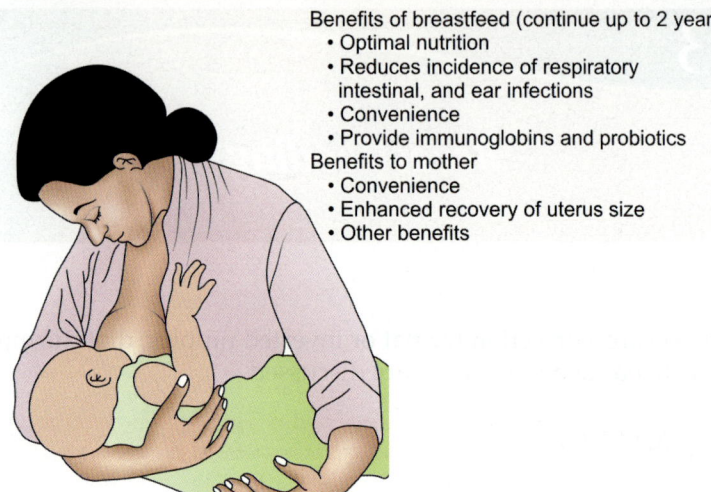

Benefits of breastfeed (continue up to 2 years)
- Optimal nutrition
- Reduces incidence of respiratory intestinal, and ear infections
- Convenience
- Provide immunoglobins and probiotics

Benefits to mother
- Convenience
- Enhanced recovery of uterus size
- Other benefits

Fig. 3.2: Breastfeeding position. (Mother in sitting position and baby's head raised)

B. BREAST AND NIPPLES

Mother should discuss with obstetrician to check/scan the breasts, mainly the nipples—in case of flat or inverted nipples baby is denied the right way of suction. The normal, flat and inverted (inverted nipples are due to short ligament, which pulls the nipple inwards) shapes of the nipples are shown below (Fig. 3.3).

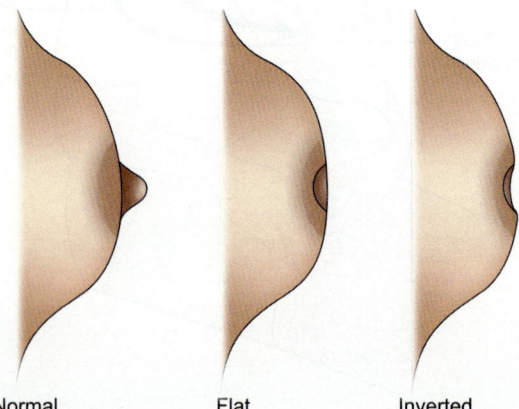

Normal   Flat   Inverted

Fig. 3.3: Normal and abnormal shapes of breast nipples, i.e. flat and inverted

These nipple defects can be corrected by Syringe Method. Contact your pediatrician or a nurse who has worked in newborn care unit (Fig. 3.4).

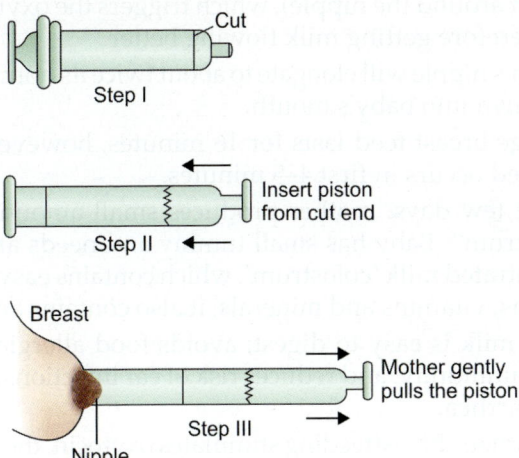

Step I — Cut

Step II — Insert piston from cut end

Step III — Breast, Nipple, Mother gently pulls the piston

Fig. 3.4: Simple technique to form the breast nipple by suction technique by a syringe

On average nipple has 9 outlets; both breasts produce same milk; baby may prefer one of them. Once the baby attaches to breast, more milk is formed.

Milk leaking: Happens right before feeding or when baby cries. You may put some sterile pad inside bra and change pad and bra often.

Sore nipples: Vigorous sucking or improper latching on, may cause sore or cracked nipples. Try new position while feeding and air dry your nipples. *Rub your own breast milk/colostrums around the nipples.*

Breast pain: Tingling is a normal experience of your body for releasing milk. Use warm or cold compresses on your breast during feedings.

Baby needs to take in the entire nipple and a large part of the areola in order for a good latch and good milk transfer. The nipple should touch the soft palate in baby's mouth.

With a good latch like this one, it is almost impossible for mom to have sore or broken nipples as baby's teeth are far away from the nipple and the nipple is protected by the soft palate (Fig. 3.2).

This latch will also ensure that baby is stimulating the areola (dark part around the nipple), which triggers the oxytocin hormone, therefore getting milk flowing better.

A mom's nipple will elongate to about twice its normal length when drawn into baby's mouth.

1. Average breast feed lasts for 16 minutes, however around 90% feed occurs in first 4–5 minutes.

2. In first few days, mother produces small amount of milk "colostrum". Baby has small tummy and needs are met by concentrated milk 'colostrum', which contains easy to digest proteins, vitamins and minerals; it also contains antibodies.

3. Breast milk is easy to digest; avoids food allergies; boosts baby's immunity, and reduces risk of ear infections, allergies and diarrhea.

4. For mothers, breastfeeding stimulates oxytocin, the hormone that causes uterus to contract and return to normal size; lowers your fat stores, and prevents breast and ovarian cancer.

During lactation, women do not need to wash their nipples with soap. The use of soap may cause drying and cracking of nipples. Daily bathing is encouraged; the nipples do not need to be washed after each feed or prior to a feed. Prior to each feed, some gentle massage may be helpful in stimulating the milk ejection reflex.

After each nursing, the expression and application of a few drops of breast milk onto the nipple will help protect the skin and heal abrasions. The use of most nipple creams is not recommended. Milk expression either by hand or with a pump should never be painful or should never cause trauma to the breast. Women may benefit from the additional *breast support* provided by a properly fitted nursing bra. Many women will elect to use breast pads if they leak milk. *These breast pads should not have plastic liners.*

Exercises which help tone and strengthen the underlying chest muscles will help maintain breast shape. Sagging and drooping of a breast is a result of age, gravity and the influence of pregnancy. Lactation alone does not cause changes in breast.

SUCKING

- Establishes when mother pick's up her baby
- Newborn must approach/latch onto and manipulate the nipple
- Within a few days full term infant comprises short bursts at least 30 sucks/min with coordinated swallowing
- Sucking liquid – chewing – mixing with saliva
- Sucking creates overall stimulation of its mouth
- Flow of milk in pharynx switches from the non-nutritive mode to nutritive mode
- Structure and resiliency of the nipple/taste, smell are conditioning stimuli
- Gastric filling stops sucking

C. FOOD DURING BREASTFEEDING

Remember, there is no need to go on a special diet while you are breastfeeding. Simply focus on making healthy choices—and you and your baby will reap the rewards.

If you are breastfeeding, you are giving your baby nutrients that will promote his or her optimal growth and brain growth and development.

You need extra calories while breastfeeding—*Understand the basics of breastfeeding nutrition.*

You need to eat a little more—about an additional 400 to 500 calories a day—to keep up your energy. To get these extra calories, opt for nutrient-rich choices, from the core food groups cooked in tasteful manner with peanut oil, a banana or an apple, and 8 ounces (about 227 gm) of fat-free yogurt.

Opt for a variety of whole grains as well as fruits and vegetables. Wash your fruits and vegetables to reduce exposure to pesticide residue.

Eating a variety of different foods while breastfeeding will change the flavor of your breast milk. This will expose your baby to different tastes, which might help him or her more easily accept solid foods during weaning.

To make sure you and your baby are getting all of the vitamins you need, continue to take a daily prenatal vitamin and calcium until you wean your baby.

D. FLUID WHILE BREASTFEEDING

It is important for breastfeeding moms to stay hydrated. Be sure to drink frequently, preferably before you feel thirsty, and to drink more if your urine appears dark yellow.

Have a glass of water nearby when you breastfeed your baby—or aim to drink at least eight glasses of water or other liquids a day.

Juices, drinks, can contribute to weight gain.

Too much caffeine can be troublesome. Limit yourself to not more than 2 to 3 cups of caffeinated drinks a day. Caffeine in your breast milk might agitate your baby or interfere with your baby's sleep.

Foods and drinks to be limited while breastfeeding.

Vegetarian Diet in Breastfeeding

If you follow a vegetarian diet, you likely already know the importance of choosing foods that will give you the nutrients you need. This is especially important during breastfeeding.

Choose Foods Rich in Iron, Protein and Calcium

During breastfeeding, make an extra effort to ensure that your diet includes plenty of these nutrients.

Good sources of **iron** include dried beans, peas, lentils, enriched cereals, whole-grain products, dark leafy green vegetables, and dried fruits. To help your body absorb iron, eat iron-rich foods in combination with foods high in vitamin C, such as citrus fruits, mango or tomatoes. Cooking in cast iron utensils adds extra iron.

For **protein,** consider eggs and dairy products or plant sources, such as soy products and meat substitutes, legumes, lentils, nuts, seeds, and whole grains.

Good sources of **calcium** include dairy products and dark green vegetables. Other options include calcium-enriched and fortified products, such as juices, cereals, soy milk, soy yogurt, etc.

Consider Supplements

You take a *daily vitamin B₁₂ + iron + folic acid tablet and calcium with vitamin D supplement.* If you do not eat enough vitamin D-fortified foods—such as cow's milk and some cereals —and you have limited sun exposure (as in case of crowded flats/winter months), you might need vitamin D supplements. Your baby needs vitamin D to absorb calcium and phosphorus. Too little vitamin D can cause *rickets*, a softening and weakening of bones. Vitamin B_{12} is found almost exclusively in animal products, so it can be difficult to get enough in some vegetarian diets. Vitamin B_{12} is essential for your baby's brain development and maintenance of hemoglobin.

Fish

Seafood can be a great source of protein and omega-3 fatty acids. Most seafoods contain mercury, which through breast milk can pose a risk to a baby's developing nervous system. You can choose seafood that is low in mercury, such as shrimp, salmon, canned light tuna and catfish. Avoid seafood that is high in mercury, including shark, swordfish, king mackerel and tilefish.

If you eat fish from local waters, pay attention to local fish advisories. If advice is not available, limit fish from local waters to 170 gm a week and do not eat other fish that week (specially for mothers in coastal area and Bengal).

Diet Causing Allergic Reaction in Baby

Certain foods or drinks in your diet could cause your baby to become irritable or have an allergic reaction.

If your baby becomes fussy or develops a rash, diarrhea or congestion soon after nursing, consult your baby's doctor. These signs could indicate a food allergy.

If you suspect that something in your diet might be making your baby a little fussier than usual, avoid the food or drink for up to a week to see if it makes a difference in your baby's behavior. Consider eliminating dairy products or other allergenic foods or ingredients, such as:

- Cow's milk
- Eggs

- Peanuts
- Nuts
- Wheat
- Soy
- Fish

Smoking

In case you are addicted to smoking, it is advised that you give up the habit before you conceive.

Smoking during pregnancy has also been linked to sudden infant death syndrome, or SIDS. Researchers have found that kids and teens born to smoking moms were more likely to take psychiatric medications than the moms who had not smoked (*see* Reuters health story of August 26, 2011.) Tobacco smoke contains toxic chemicals. When you smoke, these chemicals are absorbed into your blood and passed to your baby through the umbilical cord. Carbon monoxide replaces the oxygen in your blood, reducing the amount of oxygen available to your baby. Nicotine causes your blood vessels to narrow, reducing the flow of blood through the umbilical cord and the amount of nutrients being provided to your baby. It also reduces your baby's ability to exercise their chest muscles in preparation for breathing after birth.

Certain foods and drinks deserve caution while you are breastfeeding. For example:

Alcohol

There is no level of alcohol in breast milk that is considered safe for a baby.

Alcohol is Dangerous in Pregnancy

When a pregnant woman drinks alcohol, so does her unborn baby through placenta.

Your liver works hard to break down the alcohol in your blood. But your baby's liver is too small to do the same.

Drinking alcohol during pregnancy can cause miscarriage, stillbirth, and a range of lifelong disorders, known as fetal alcohol spectrum disorders (FASDs). Children with FASDs might have the following characteristics and behaviors:

- Abnormal facial features, such as a smooth ridge between the nose and upper lip (this ridge is called the philtrum)
- Small head size
- Shorter-than-average height
- Low body weight
- Poor coordination
- Hyperactive behavior
- Difficulty paying attention
- Poor memory
- Difficulty in school (especially in maths)
- Learning disabilities
- Speech and language delays
- Intellectual disability or low IQ
- Poor reasoning and judgment skills
- Sleep and sucking problems as a baby
- Vision or hearing problems
- Problems with the heart, kidney, or bones

Nguyen, T. Coppens, J and Riley, E. (2011). 'Prenatal alcohol exposure, FAS and FASD: An introduction.' In E.P Rilley, S Clarren, J Weinberg and E Jonsson (Eds). *Fetal Alcohol Spectrum Disorder: Management and Policy perspectives of FASD* (pp 1–13). Weinheim, Wiley-VCH Verlay GmbH & Co. KGaA

*It is recommended not to consume alcohol
(Center Disease Control, USA)*

Caffeine

Avoid drinking more than 2 to 3 cups of caffeinated drinks a day. Remember, caffeine in your breast milk might agitate your baby or interfere with your baby's sleep.

Caffeine is harmful: The UK Food Standards Agency recommended daily dose of caffeine in pregnancy—200 mg, i.e. 2 cups of instant coffee, two mugs of tea, six cans of coca-cola or four 50 g bars of chocolate. A coffee from a cafe may be stronger, it could contain more than 200 mg caffeine.

The Norwegian mother and child study (more than 59,000 pregnant women have taken part in the research over 10 years) shows, that caffeine reduces the birth weight. Babies with lower birth weight have an increased risk of diabetes, high blood pressure and heart disease in adulthood (The Guardian, Monday, 25th Feb. 2013).

E. BREASTFEEDING STRUGGLE

If you are struggling, ask your pediatrician for help. Breast milk is the ideal food for babies—and the best way to keep a baby healthy—proper nutrition and hydration are absolutely essential.

Does Infant Formula Pose any Risks to a Baby?

Commercial infant formulas do not contain the immunity-boosting elements of breast milk. For most babies, breast milk is also easier to digest than formula.

A baby who has special nutritional needs might require a special formula (lactose intolerance).

Combination of Breastfeeding and Formula Feeding

Exclusive breastfeeding is typically recommended for the first six months after birth. Some working mothers are able to successfully combine breastfeeding and formulafeeding—especially after breastfeeding has been well established.

Breastfeeding is Rarely Contraindicated

- Recommend an acceptable alternative to breastfeeding for mothers who are HIV-infected.
- Advise that most medications are compatible with breast feeding. Take a case-by-case approach when a mother is using medications or drugs.

F. POINTS FOR BREASTFEEDING POSITION

Choose a comfortable chair with arm rests, and use pillows—lots of them—to lend extra support to your back and arms, or most comfortable squatting position to feed the baby—stick a few pillows under your feet too, to avoid bending towards your baby (Fig. 3.5).

Nursing position—be sure to bring your baby to your breast.

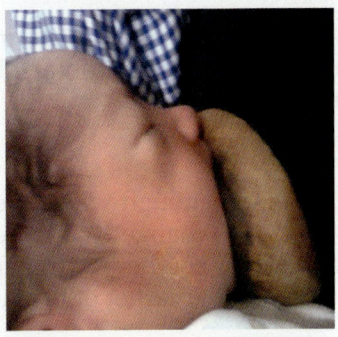 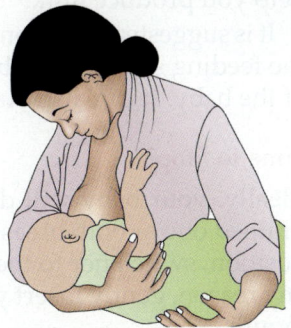

Fig. 3.5: Baby on breast, mother in sitting position with baby head on arm

Support Your Breasts

Your breasts get bigger and heavier during lactation. As you nurse, use your free hand to support your breast.

It is important to keep your fingers at least 2 inches behind the nipple and areola so that your baby does not suck on them instead.

Support Your Baby

Feeling comfortable and secure will help your baby nurse happily and efficiently. Use your arm and hand, plus pillows, to support your baby's head, neck, back, and hips and keep them in a straight line.

Vary Your Routine

Find a nursing position that you find most comfortable. Many women find that the best way to avoid getting 'clogged milk ducts' is to regularly alternate breastfeeding holds. Because each hold puts pressure on a different part of your nipple, you may avoid getting "sore nipples" too.

Alternate breast, at each feed.

Relax, then Nurse

Take a few deep breaths, close your eyes, and think peaceful, calming thoughts. Keep a tall, cool glass of water, milk, or juice on hand to drink while you breastfeed—staying hydrated will help you produce milk.

It is suggested to put on some instrumental music CD during the feeding session. It is believed to stimulate left frontal lobe of the baby. It can also build conditioning reflex.

Time to Stop?

Ideally, your baby will decide she's had enough when she's drained one or both breasts. If you need to change your baby's position, switch her to the other breast, or end her feeding for any reason, gently insert your finger into the corner of his/her mouth.

G. BURPING

After breastfeeding, try to burp the baby. If your baby does not burp after 10 minutes, then baby most likely does not have a wind. After drinking from each breast, try to burp the baby. *If your baby spits up a lot, you should burp the baby more often* (Fig. 3.6).

Burp the baby while baby is sitting up on your leg, leaning forward with your hand under baby's chin for support, while the other hand pats baby gently on the back.

Walking while burping your baby will also help get rid of the winds and helps calm baby.

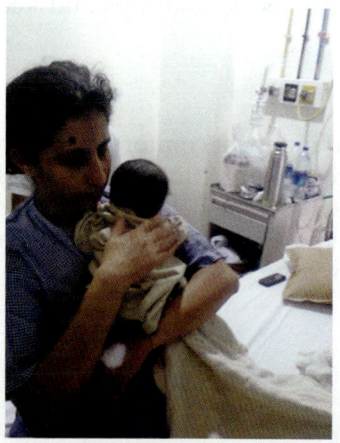 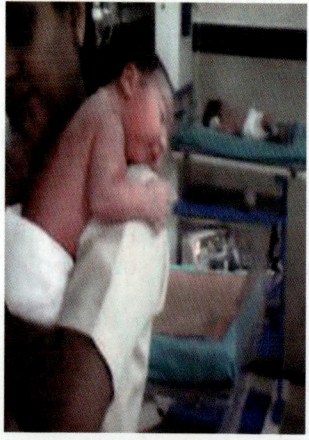

Fig. 3.6: Burping positions after breastfeeding

Breastfeeding mothers can avoid their babies from swallowing air by keeping them in an upright position (45° angle).

H. LYING POSITION AFTER FEEDING

Raise the head by 45° by using two pillows and put one pillow on either side (Figs 3.7 and 3.8).

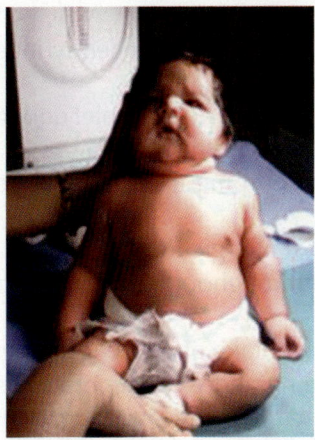

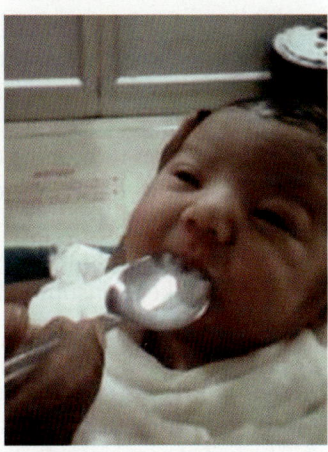

Fig. 3.7: Put 2 pillows under head and one pillow on either side to hold baby in upright position after feeding

Fig. 3.8: Spoonfeeding (head is raised)

BREASTFEEDING — HOW LONG?

A landmark decision to protect, promote and support breastfeeding was taken in 54th World Health Assembly in 2001, giving rise to a Global Public Health recommendation for exclusive breastfeeding for first six months of life, complementary feeding with home based safe and nutritious foods to start at six months of age and continued breastfeeding up to the age of two years and beyond.

Correct Norms for Infant and Young Child Feeding

- Initiation of breastfeeding immediately after birth—preferably within 30 minutes.

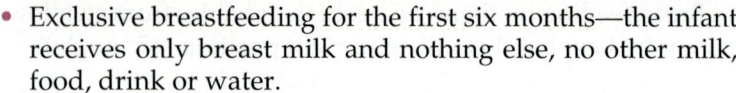

- Exclusive breastfeeding for the first six months—the infant receives only breast milk and nothing else, no other milk, food, drink or water.
- Appropriate and adequate complementary feeding—from six months of age while continuing breastfeeding.
- Continued breastfeeding up to the age of two years or beyond.

Key Notes

- In late pregnancy, get your nipples checked, if needed syringe correction to ensure proper breastfeeding.
- Maintain balanced diet and calcium + iron folate tablet during active lactation (6 months exclusive breastfeeding).
- Position of the baby in lactation, burping and postfeed be upright(head raised).
- Mother should not take any known allergic food.
- Do not smoke; consume alcohol throughout pregnancy and lactation.
- Caffeine is restricted by controlling intake of coffee/tea/coke.

Current status in India: Infant feeding and weaning practices in India continue to demonstrate that a significant number of infants do not receive colostrum (62.8% as per National Family Health Survey, NFHS-2), though breastfeeding is universal and continued for a longer period. In NFHS-3 (2005–06):

a. There is improving trend for breastfeeding within first hour of birth (23.4%).
b. Exclusive breastfeeding up to 5 months (46.3%).
c. However, weaning for semisolids is delayed (55.8% only in 6–9 months of age).

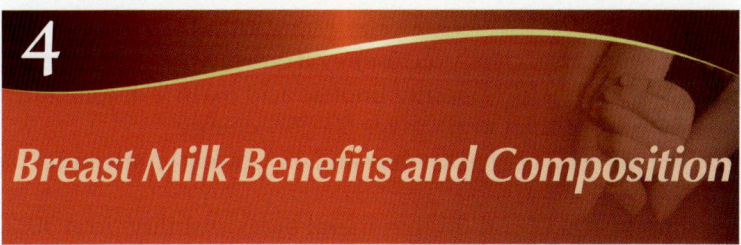

4

Breast Milk Benefits and Composition

We will discuss unique composition of breast milk and immune properties. Lactation has benefits for mother as well as infant.

A. IMPORTANT FACTS ABOUT FIRST BREAST MILK CALLED COLOSTRUM

- Rich in protective factors
- Facilitates establishment of bifido flora in the digestive tract
- Yellow color is due to –β carotene
- It flows for first 3 days
- Rich source of antibodies
- Rich in antidiarrheal factors
- High mineral content
- Higher concentration of fat soluble vitamins, minerals and electrolytes—Na, K, Cl than mature milk.

Interesting Facts About Colostrum on GI Tract

1. Colostrum facilitates the establishment of bifidus flora in the digestive tract.
2. Colostrum also facilitates the passage of meconium.

Describe Transitional Milk

Major changes in breast milk composition occur on **transition** from colostrum to mature milk between 3 and 10th day.

B. BREAST MILK—FOOD VALUES AND COMPOSITION

From 10th day onwards MATURE BREAST MILK: 58–72 kcal/ 100 ml; low protein 0.9–1.2 gm/100 ml; high in cystine and taurine; low cystine:methionine ratio.

Breast Milk Contains

- Carbohydrates (chiefly lactose)—7.0 gm; gives 40–45% energy.
- Fats—3.8 gm; EFA mainly linoleic acid (6–16% of total fatty acids; 3% of total kcal); gives 50–55% energy.
- Proteins—1.2 gm (60% whey and 40% casein) contribute 7% energy.
- Minerals—0.21 gm (high mineral bioavailability; iron 50%, zinc 39% and calcium 75%); low in phosphorus.
- Vitamins—vitamin A and thiamine.

  Note: There are around 200 recognized constituents in breast milk.

Other Important Factors Present in Breast Milk Besides Nutrients

a. Enzymes—amylases(starches); lipases(fats), and proteases (proteins).
b. Protective factors:
   i. *Lactoferrin*—protects against gastrointestinal infection in breast fed infants, inhibits the growth of iron dependent bacteria.

      Note: Giving extra iron to neonates inactivates lactoferrin.
   ii. *Lysozyme*—antimicrobial enzyme. Contributes to the development and maintenance of good intestinal flora of the breastfed infant.
   iii. *Immunoglobulins*—proteins synthesized by the immune system include all known antibodies. sIgA protects against food allergens (allergy) and microbial antigens (infection). The principle Ig in human milk: sIgA is 17 times in colostrum than mature milk. It is resistant to protein splitting enzymes and present in the intestines of breastfed infants.
   iv. *Bifidus factor*—growth factor for bifido bacteria, do not require the presence of intestinal enzymes for activation. It is responsible for the implantation and proliferation of bifido bacteria in the breastfed infant's intestine.
   v. *Immune cells*—
      - Lymphocytes: Synthesize IgA antibody.
      - Macrophages: Phagocytosis (killing of bacteria); and production of lysozyme and lactoferrin.
      - Leucocytes: Phagocytosis and microbial killing.

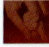

vi. *Hormones in the breast milk*—there are 16 different types of hormones in breast milk. Some of the hormones are thyroxine, prolactin and insulin.

Other Benefits of Breast Milk

- A close mother/infant bond
- Less risk of vaginal bleeds
- Quicker return to prepregnancy weight
- Reduction of natural fertility

Breast milk has deficiencies of vitamins K, B_{12} and D.

NORMAL BREASTFED INFANT OF A WELL-NOURISHED MOTHER

- Receives all vitamins, except K, D and B_{12}
- Vitamin K—**Hemorrhagic** disease of newborn
- Vitamin D—extremely low content, 22 or < 25 IU/l. Need 400 IU/day (RDA); if limited exposure to sunlight—**RICKETS**.
- **Vitamin B_{12}**—vegetarian mothers have low breast milk; particularly in lacto vegetarians—**megaloblastic anemia**.

ENERGY REQUIREMENTS FOR TERM INFANT

- First month of life—115 kcal/kg/d–rapid and vigorous fat deposit
- By 6 months of life—85 kcal/kg/d
- By end of first year—100 kcal/kg/d
- By the time infant wt. doubles birth weight ~4–5 months; fat in body trebles (25% of the total body weight), while during 6–12 months fat deposit is 500 gm only

Important nutrients for infants include carbohydrates, protein, fat, vitamins and minerals. Breast milk generally contains sufficient amounts of required nutrients for infants, with the exception of vitamin D and iron, which are low in breast milk. However, iron absorption from breast milk is higher. Therefore, a well-nourished nonanemic mother will meet the iron needs in first 6 months of life. Omega-3 fatty acids are important for your infant's brain development. The

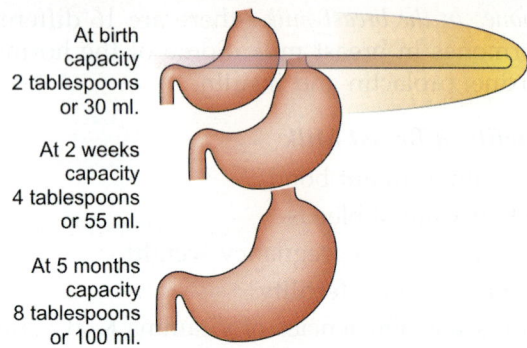

At birth
capacity
2 tablespoons
or 30 ml.

At 2 weeks
capacity
4 tablespoons
or 55 ml.

At 5 months
capacity
8 tablespoons
or 100 ml.

Fig. 4.1: Baby's stomach—actual size

Institute of Medicine (IOM), USA encourages infants up to 6 months of age to consume at least 60 gm of carbohydrates, 9.1 gm of protein, 31 gm of total fat and 500 milligrams of omega-3s each day and for ages 7 to 12 months to consume at least 95 gm of carbohydrates, 11 gm of protein, 30 gm of total fat and 500 mg of omega-3s everyday.

How much to feed? Infant's stomach measures around the size of baby's left fist, so do not force feed (Fig. 4.1).

Key Notes

- Colostrum (milk in first 3–4 days) and breast milk have **ideal** nutritive values for infant growth, brain development and establishment of immune properties.
- However, breast milk is **poor** in vitamin K— (hemorrhagic disease of newborn bleeding tendency at birth), low vitamin D (rickets), and low vitamin B_{12} (megaloblastic anemia).

5

Essentials for Baby Care
(Must inculcate during later pregnancy)

Discussion stresses strict hygiene by mother/ baby care giver, diaper and dress, baby bath (when to start), how to give.

A. MOTHER SHOULD OBSERVE STRICT HYGIENE

Clip off her nails every third day.

Minimize wearing of rings or ornaments in hands.

Wash hands with soap and water before handling the baby.

Should brush/paste teeth after every meal, at least 3 times, last being before bed.

Change clothes 2 times a day, preferably take bath.

Comb hair and tie; should not touch again and again to avoid infection of hands.

If mother has any doubt of illness, then get checked and treated.

Do inform your pediatrician about the medicines you are taking; as some medicines pass in breast milk and can harm the baby.

B. DIAPERS AND DRESS FOR BABY

Stitch simple soft cotton diapers in dozens, preferably out of washed old soft cotton cloth (saree). These can be reused after washing/drying in sunlight and ironing (Fig. 5.1).

Baby diaper should be changed after urination and/or defecation. It should be cleaned or stored outside the baby's room. Wash these with good quality detergent as chemicals if used can cause skin allergy/burn.

Presently colorful fancy baby dresses are in market. Choose/ prepare at home by stitching soft cotton (poplin) shirts without

43

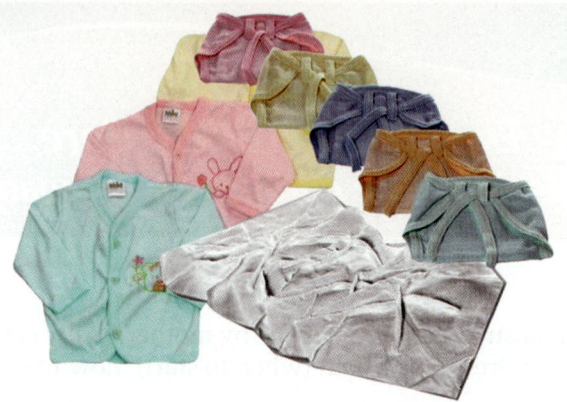

Fig. 5.1: The simple designs for dresses and diapers

collar, front open (coverable with string or buttons). These should also be washed with good quality detergents with plenty of water, sun dry and iron. Note that baby dresses should be simple; do not use decorative lining. Dresses should be light colored. Yellow color dress in first 3 weeks is avoided as some babies develop physiological jaundice. The yellow color dress may interfere in judgement of jaundice.

C. BABY BATH

For our country, India, better use RO filtered water for sponge cleaning and bath.

Bathing a slippery newborn can be a difficult practice. There is no need to give your newborn a bath everyday. In fact, *bathing your baby more than several times a week will dry out skin.* If you are quick with clean diapers and burp clothes, you have already cleaned the parts that really need attention, i.e. the face, neck and diaper area.

Bath time: That is up to you. Choose a time when you are more free or likely to be uninterrupted. Some parents opt for morning baths, when their babies are alert and ready to enjoy the experience. Others prefer to make baby baths part of a calming bedtime ritual.

A baby bath does not necessarily need to be done in a tub of water. The American Academy of Pediatrics recommends sponge baths until the umbilical cord stump falls off, which might take up to three weeks. If you would like to give your baby a sponge bath, you will need:

- A warm place with a flat surface. A bathroom or kitchen counter, changing table or firm bed will work. Even a blanket or towel on the floor is OK, if it is warm enough.
- A soft towel or changing pad. Spread it out for your baby to lie on.
- Always keep one hand on your baby. On a changing table, use the safety strap as well.
- A sink or shallow plastic basin to hold the water. Run warm water into the basin or sink. Check the water temperature with your hand to make sure it is not too hot.
- Gather a wash cloth, a towel—preferably with a built-in hood—cotton balls, mild baby shampoo, mild moisturizing soap, baby wipes, a clean diaper and a change of clothes.

When you are ready to begin the sponge bath, undress your baby and wrap in a towel. Lay your baby on his or her back on the towel or pad you have prepared. Wet the wash cloth, wring out excess water and wipe your baby's face. There is no need to use soap. Use a damp cotton ball or clean cotton cloth to wipe each eyelid, from the inside to the outside corner. When you are ready to clean your baby's body, filtered water is usually OK. If your baby is smelly or dirty, use a mild moisturizing soap. We have been recommending Dove/Pears/Cetaphil/ Teddybar soaps. **There is no need to use soap daily for a baby bath. In fact, filtered water is fine for newborns.** *Avoid bubble bath and scented soaps.*

Pay special attention to creases under the arms, behind the ears, around the neck and in the diaper area. Also wash between your baby's fingers and toes. To keep your baby warm, expose only the parts you are washing.

Most newborns *do not need lotion* after a bath. The best way to prevent rashes is to dry inside your baby's folds of skin after each bath. If you choose to use lotion, pick one that is hypo-allergenic.

Remember, though, safety is the most important considera-tion—not necessarily the type of tub. Gather the same supplies you would use for a sponge bath and a cup of rinsing water ahead of time so that you can keep one hand on the baby at all times. Never leave your baby alone near or in the water.

You will need only 2 to 3 inches level or 5–7 cm of warm water (check with your hand) for a baby bath (temperature 30–32°C). To keep your baby warm, pour warm water over his or her body throughout the bath.

Always check the water temperature with your hand before bathing your baby. Be sure the room is comfortably warm, too. A wet baby can be easily chilled.

A secure hold will help your baby feel comfortable—and stay safe—in the tub. Use one of your hands to support your baby's head and the other to hold and guide your baby's body into the water, feet first. Support your baby's head and torso with your arm and hand. Wrap your arm under your baby's back, grasping your baby firmly under the armpit. When you clean your baby's back and buttocks, lean him or her forward on your arm. Continue to grasp your baby under the armpit.

Most parents start with the baby's face and move on to dirtier parts of the body. Wash inside skin folds, and rinse the genitals carefully.

Wash your newborn's hair, if it seems dirty or your baby develops cradle cap—a common condition characterized by scaly patches on the scalp.

Supporting your baby's head and shoulders with your free hand, gently massage a drop of mild baby shampoo into your baby's scalp. Rinse the shampoo with a damp wash cloth or directly under the faucet, cupping one hand across your baby's forehead to keep suds out of his or her eyes. If your baby has cradle cap, loosen the scales with a soft-bristled baby brush or toothbrush before rinsing off the shampoo.

Massage Oil

Our studies have shown that plain til oil (sesame oil) is good, experience confirms that plain coconut oil is a good choice too.

Key Notes

- Mothers should learn/practice strict hygienic methods in feeding; changing diapers/vomits and sponging.
- Baby bath—give full attention, feel water temperature and keep water level 5–6 cm.
- Use moisturizing soap 3–4 times a week.

Massage oil—use coconut or sesame (til) oils.

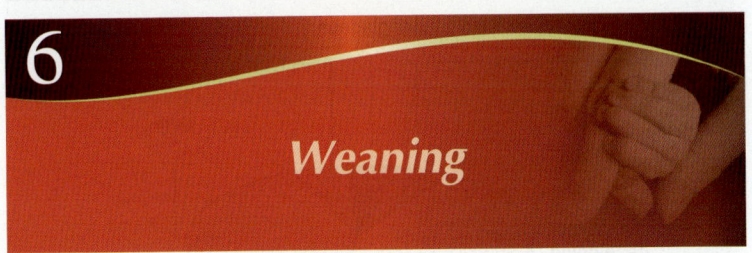

6

Weaning

The process is difficult for choice of food and hygiene mainte-nance **(sterilization of utensils and cooking—both in pressure cooker)**. The feeding techniques, first and subsequent choice of food are discussed to help the mother.

A. CURRENT STATUS

1. The infant weaning foods are inadequate in energy and/or protein, as well as micronutrients.
2. Weaning foods and feeding/cooking utensils are loaded with bacterial contamination resulting in frequent episodes of diarrhea.

These are the factors responsible for continued early mal-nutrition, which the country has failed to control as observed in the three National Family Health Surveys. Over a span of 7 years, i.e. from National Family Health Survey (NFHS)-2 (1998–99) to NFHS-3 (2005–06), there was only marginal reduc-tion in undernutrition. In 2011, an independent national survey showed that 42% children < 3 years of age are underweight (Fig. 6.1). Thus, *uncontrolled fetal malnutrition, poor initiation of breastfeeding, inadequate and delayed weaning, and contamination in food and water* demand urgency to develop affordable hygienic weaning foods at family level, education to clean utensils, timely weaning and available potable chlorinated water to prevent and control malnutrition.

Weaning

It is the process of gradually introducing foods other than breast milk in a child's feeding schedule. *This process starts when any food besides mother's milk is introduced in the child's diet and is*

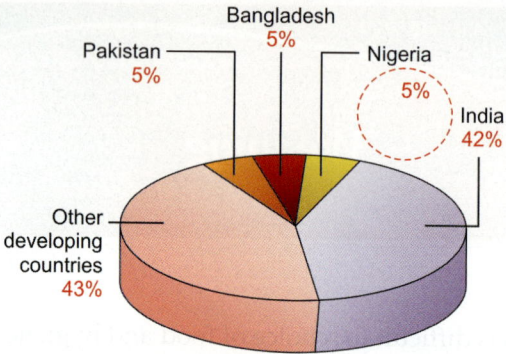

Fig. 6.1: India's contribution to the underweight burden children under-5 years of age

---

BMJ March 2013 Children 0–59 Months

- 30% of global < 5 yr deaths are in India, more than any other country
- Every minute 3 children < 5 year die
- 50% are malnourished and 70% are anemic
- Malnutrition—all India
- RURAL Unwt = 45.6; stunted = 50.7 Ws = 20.7
- URBAN Unwt = 32.7; stunted = 39.6 Ws = 16.9
- In addition, 67,000 women die of puerperal sepsis/year–a shame
- Unwt = underweight;
- Ws = wasted

---

completed only when the child has been entirely off the breast. The introduction of supplementary foods not only ensures the fulfillment of nutritional requirements, but also introduces the child gradually to the normal family eating patterns. Infants are at greatest risk of **diarrhea** when foods other than breast milk are first given. This is because, during weaning, infants are being exposed to food-borne germs for the first time and they lose the protection of breast milk which has anti-infective properties. High levels of contamination are often found in animal milk and traditional weaning foods, especially prepared cereal gruels (rice, pulse, and semolina). *Escherichia coli,* which causes at least 25 percent of all diarrheas, is commonly found in weaning foods. Feeding bottles and rubber teats, which are particularly difficult to clean, and are often breeding grounds for germs. **Ideally clean with liquid detergent and use pressure cooker to sterilize—bottles, nipple, bowl, spoons, etc.**

B. STERILIZATION OF FEEDING UTENSILS

There is need for infants older than 6 months to receive more than just breast milk in order to grow well, balanced against the risk of getting sufficient energy, proteins, vitamins and minerals, and the meals being prepared hygienically. It is important for health personnel/TV media and pediatricians to teach the family. There is scope to work with local communities to identify and encourage safe weaning practices and to improve infant's nutrition to increase their resistance to infections and prevent diarrhea. Unfortunately, shining India fails to provide clean water supply, and electricity for water filters to work (Fig. 6.2).

C. HYGIENIC PREPARATION AND STORAGE OF COMPLEMENTARY FOODS

To prevent contamination, personal hygiene plays an important role in feeding infants. *If cleanliness is not observed, complementary feeding may do more harm than good to the child by introducing infections to the infant.* It is, therefore, important that all foods prepared for young infants are handled in a way that they are free from any germs.

Some of the considerations while preparing foods for infants are as under:

- Hands should be washed with soap and water before handling the food as germs that cannot be seen in dirty hands can be passed on to the food.

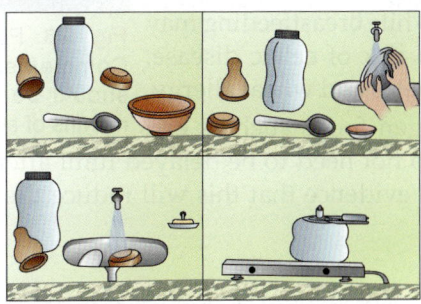

Fig. 6.2: Sterilization of baby feeding utensils in pressure cooker

- Utensils used should be scrubbed, washed well, **if possible sterilized in pressure cooker** and kept covered.
- Cooking kills most germs. The food prepared for infants should be cooked preferably in **pressure cooker** properly so as to destroy harmful bacteria present, if any.
- After cooking, handle the food as little as possible and keep it in a covered container protected from dust and flies.
- Cooked food should not be kept for more than one to two hours in hot climate. Store them in refrigerator temperature.

The hands of both mother and child should be washed before feeding the child.

D. RECOMMENDATIONS FOR WEANING 2008

The European Society for Pediatric Gastroenterology, Hepatology and Nutrition and the North American Society for Pediatric Gastroenterology, Hepatology and Nutrition reviewed the literature on complementary feeding for healthy term infants in 2008 and recommended that:

- Exclusive breastfeeding for around 6 months is a desirable goal.
- Weaning onto solid foods should begin by 6 months but not before 4 months.
- Breastfeeding continues throughout weaning particularly the early stages.

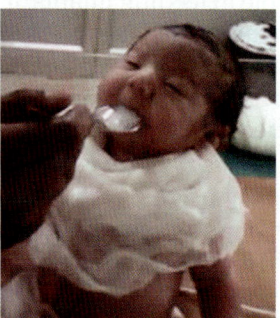

- Introducing gluten* between 4 and 7 months while breastfeeding may reduce the risk of celiac disease, type 1 diabetes and wheat allergy.

Fig. 6.3: Position for milk. Complementary feeding should be started at six months of age

- High allergen foods such as egg and fish do not need to be delayed until after 6 months as there is no evidence that this will reduce the likelihood of allergies.

---

*Foods containing gluten are wheat, rye, barley and oats. These cereals are present in bread, wheat flour, some breakfast cereal and toasts.

- The purpose of complementary feeding is to complement the breast milk and make certain that the young child continues to have enough energy, protein and other nutrients to grow normally.
- Adequate complementary feeding from six months of age while continuing breastfeeding is extremely important for sustaining growth and development of the infant.
- Active feeding styles for complementary feeding are also important.
- Appropriate feeding styles can provide significant learning opportunities through responsive care giver interaction, enhancing brain development in the most crucial first three years.
- It is important that breastfeeding is continued up to the age of two years or beyond as it provides useful amount of energy, good quality protein and other nutrients.

E. AGE OF INTRODUCTION OF SOLID FOODS

- It is recommended that healthy term infants need no nutrition other than breast milk or formula milk until six months (26 weeks) of age.
- In case of working mothers, babies may be ready for solids from 4–5 months of age. Each baby should be assessed on his/her needs for solids individually (Fig. 6.4).

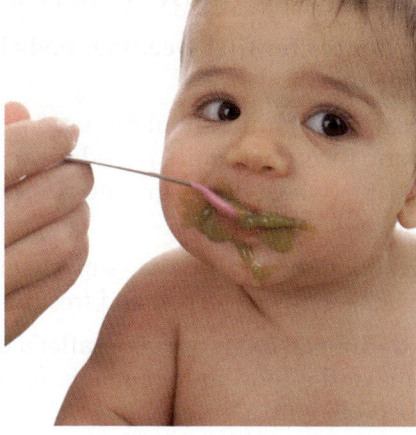

Fig. 6.4: Baby in sitting position for semisolids

- Premature babies must be assessed individually for their readiness for solids.

F. SIGNS OF READINESS TO FEED (WEANING)

Term babies are born between 37 and 42 weeks of gestation, they grow and develop at different rates. This means some infants will be ready to begin weaning early, in postnatal age between > 4–6 months. Mothers usually begin weaning large infants and male infants earlier than others.

In practice, the *developmental signs that suggest that an infant is ready to accept solid foods are:*

- *Putting toys and other objects in the mouth*
- *Chewing fists*
- *Watching others with interest when they are eating*
- *Seeming hungry between milk feeds or demanding feeds more often even though larger milk feeds have been offered*

These developmental signs are generally seen between 4 and 6 months and this seems to be the best time to start solids because from this age infants learn to accept new tastes and textures relatively quickly.

G. FIRST AND AGE APPROPRIATE FOOD FOR THE BABY

The workable choices for first weaning foods in our culture are discussed below:

The **staple cereal** of the family should be used to make the first food for an infant. Rice, dal (lentil), porridge can be made with suji (semolina), atta (wheat flour), ground rice, ragi, millet, etc. by using a little milk.

Mixed foods like khichidi, dalia, suji kheer, upma, idli, dokhla, bhaat-bhaji, halwa, etc. soft and freshly prepared.

Sometimes traditional foods are given after a little modification so as to make the food more suitable for the child. For instance, mashed idli with a little oil and dal is a good complementary food for the infant.

Similarly, rice can be made more nutritious by adding some cooked dal or vegetable to it. Khichidi (mixture of rice+dal) can be made more nutritious by adding one or two green vegetables in it while cooking.

Fruits like banana, papaya, chikoo, mango, etc. could be given at this age in a mashed form.

Vegetables like tomato, carrot or mixed vegetable soup or mashed green vegetables.

Dahi/yogurt separately or as mixed in food.

Modified Family Food

- In most families, there is a cereal preparation in the form of roti or rice and a pulse or a vegetable preparation. **For preparing a complementary food for the infant from the foods cooked for the family, a small amount of dal or vegetable preparation should be separated before adding spices to it.**

- Pieces of chapatti could be soaked in half-a-*katori* of dal and some vegetable, if available. The mixed food could be mashed well and fed to the baby after adding a little oil.

- Thus, rice or wheat preparation could be mixed with pulse and/or vegetable to make a nutritious complementary food for the infant.

- Modifying family's food is one of the most effective ways of ensuring complementary feeding of infants.

Salt and sugar must not be added to solids for infants.

How to Feed Solids (Fig. 6.5)

- The baby must be well supported in sitting position; use a reclining chair for younger babies or a high chair once they can support themselves. Some babies constantly fed in lying position and not burped **can develop ear discharge.**

- Use age-appropriate *katori*/bowls to put the food in. **The utensils should be detergent cleaned and sterilized in pressure cooker.**

- Food should be given from a **hard plastic weaning spoon** that will not crack. Do not use a metal spoon.

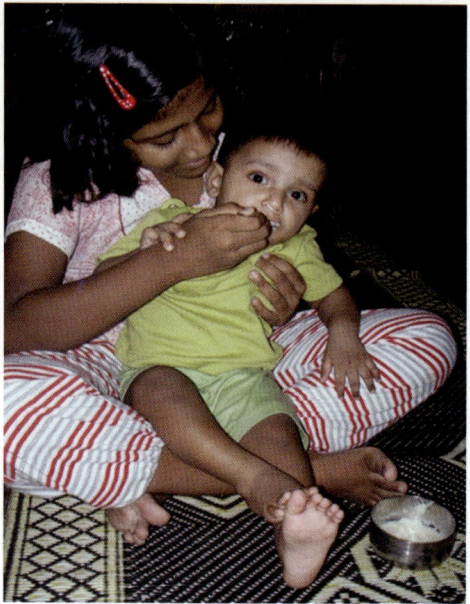

Fig. 6.5: Sister feeding the toddler

- **First weaning foods introduced are for tastes only.** A few teaspoons should be offered before one feed. If the baby likes the food's taste and flavor (acceptance), then even other foods can be given in combination of the liked food.
- Food should be of a smooth purée texture. Once the baby is happy with this, offer purée foods before a second feed, and then a third feed, gradually increasing the quantity.
- The consistency can be made thicker as the baby learns to eat. Do not move onto thicker textures too quickly. By 9–12 months of age, most healthy babies will be able to cope with minced and mashed textures.
- It is very important that babies are offered food at meal times and that eating becomes part of the daily routine.
- Allow messy play, give the baby their own spoon to feed themselves and let them use their hands. Never leave a baby alone with food.
- For older children, make sure that furniture, cutlery and crockery is age appropriate and that the dining area is a child friendly environment, without too many distractions.

Table 6.1: The type and texture of foods to be introduced at each weaning stage

Stage	Age guide	Skills to learn	New food textures to introduce
1	Begin by 6 months, but not before 4 months (17 weeks)	– taking food from a spoon – moving food from the front of the mouth to the back for swallowing – managing thicker purées and mashed food	Smooth purées, soup mashed foods (dal+rice), dahi
2	6–9 months	– thicker texture-halwa, mashed idli, poha – chewing lumps – self-feeding using hands and fingers – sipping from a cup	Mashed food with soft lumps—porridge, kheer, khichidi, banana Soft finger foods, liquids in a lidded beaker or cup
3	9–12 months	– chewing minced and chopped food – self-feeding attempts with a spoon	Semisolid foods—idli, pakora, minced and chopped family foods

In case you are just starting your baby onto solid foods, you should start your baby on puréed and liquid food (Table 6.1).

What to Feed

6–8 Months

- Breast milk or pasteurized dairy milk/formula.
- Dal water, rice water, diluted rice cereal, mashed banana diluted with baby's milk, cooked and thinly puréed fruits and vegetables. Pass the cooked fruits and vegetables through a strainer, so that there is no lump.

Later

- Gradually thicken the purées a bit. Pass the cooked fruits and vegetables through a strainer, so that there are no lumps. You can gradually introduce lumpier, mashed food as well as combination foods.
- Purée two vegetables or fruits together, e.g. apple and pear-cooked and puréed together, carrot with tomato, etc.
- Khichidi, different legumes like kidney beans, grams, black gram, chickpeas (without cover).
- Dairy—dahi or yogurt, cheese, paneer
- Tofu
  See "Food triangle" and make suitable age and development appropriate foods for this age-group with modifications in your family diet.

Note:

1. Check with your pediatrician, before introducing eggs, fish or meat to your baby's diet.
2. Whenever you introduce combination of foods, ensure that individual items have been safely introduced first. It means that if you want to give carrot and tomato soup, both carrot and tomato should have been introduced first without any issues.

8–10 Months

- Breast milk/pasteurized or formula milk.
- Dal+rice mashed, vegetables cooked for daily food (without spice).
- Bread/*roti* soaked in milk or *dal*/vegetable.
- Cooked and mashed fruits and vegetables.
- Puréed legumes , *paneer*, tofu.

What to Introduce

Different cereals, in addition to rice, semolina, ragi, whole wheat (*atta*), oats, etc.

Non-vegetarian proteins like eggs (check with your doctor before introducing eggs. Egg whites are known to cause allergic reactions in babies, so it is recommended to introduce yolks first and wait to introduce whites after 1 year), fish or chicken. Introduce your baby to lean meat which is healthier.

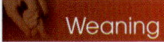

Make sure what fish or meat you introduce is well cooked, *deboned* and puréed. Follow the rule to introduce very little and only one item at a time and wait till at least 3–4 days to screen for allergies, etc.

What Not to Give

- Fish, foods allergic to mother.

10–12 Months

- Breast milk/pasteurized/formula.
- Cooked, mashed complex foods—khichidi, vegetable pulao, mixed soups, dosas, lentils, etc.

New Introduction

- You can give most of the food you are having, as long as it is not too oily, hot and spicy.

What Not to Give

- Foods brought from open, unhygienic shops/restaurants. Strictly feed homemade freshly prepared food. Cooking is done in pressure cooker.
- Honey, which can cause botulism in infants, hence it is recommended to wait till one year before giving honey.

Note: **Once you start solids, start feeding some amount of water also. It need not be more than 120–150 ml per day. Many babies suffer from constipation once they start solids. Having water will not only keep the baby hydrated, but also keep constipation at bay.**

Key Notes

- Infant weaning for semisolids in India remains faulty
  - Delayed weaning
  - Inadequacy of macro- and micronutrients
  - Bacterial contamination
  - Polluted water
    (Even in educated families, utensil cleaning remains poor)
- Faulty weaning given to poor or borderline nourished infants and further nurtured by undernourished (33%)/anemic mothers (> 80% or more).

- These infants have not received exclusive breastfeeding and share complementary feeding, mostly diluted milk.

- This sets in cycle of malnutrition with stunting and wasting with under and/or improper feeding. These children suffer with brain structural changes and functional losses.

- This is allowed to happen in India despite vibrant economy, surplus food/milk, etc.—reasons being poor management. Drinking water remains the first national priority.

Diet from 2 Years of Age (Guidelines)

Recent general dietary recommendations of the American Heart Association for those aged 2 years and older stress a diet that primarily relies on:

- Fruits and vegetables,
- Whole grains,
- Low-fat and nonfat dairy products,
- Beans, fish, and lean meat.

These general recommendations echo other recent public health dietary guidelines in emphasizing low intakes of saturated and trans fat, cholesterol, and added sugar and salt; energy intake and physical activity appropriate for the maintenance of a normal weight for height; and adequate intake of micronutrients.

- Energy (calories) should be adequate to support growth and development and to reach or maintain desirable body weight.

- Eat foods low in saturated fat, trans fat, cholesterol, salt (sodium), and added sugars.

- Keep total fat intake between 30 and 35 percent of calories for children 2 to 3 years of age and between 25 and 35 percent of calories for children and adolescents 4 to 18 years of age, with most fats coming from sources of polyunsaturated and monounsaturated fatty acids, such as fish, nuts and vegetable oils.

- Choose a variety of foods to get enough carbohydrates, protein and other nutrients.

- Eat only enough calories to maintain a healthy weight for your height and built. Be physically active for at least 60 minutes a day.

- Serve whole-grain/high-fiber roti/breads and cereals rather than refined grain products. Look for "whole grain" as the first ingredient on the food label and make at least half your grain servings whole grain. Recommended grain intake ranges from 55 gm/day for a one-year-old to 200 gm/day for a 14–18 years old boy.

- Serve a variety of fruits and vegetables daily, while limiting juice intake. Each meal should contain at least 1 fruit or vegetable. Children's recommended fruit intake ranges from 1 cup/day, between ages 1 and 3, to 2 cups for a 14–18 years old boy. Recommended vegetable intake ranges from ¾ cup a day at age one to 3 cups for a 14–18 years old boy.

- Introduce and regularly serve fish as an entrée. Avoid commercially fried fish.

- Serve fat-free and low-fat dairy foods. From ages 1–8 months, children need 2 cups of milk or its equivalent each day. Children aged 9–18 months need 3 cups.

- Do not overfeed. Estimated calories needed by children range from 900/day for a 1-year-old to 1,800 for a 14–18 years old girl and 2,200 for a 14–18 years old boy.

This eating pattern supports normal growth and development for children and adolescents, including iron and calcium needs.

These guidelines are very important for our country as low birth weight babies have risk of developing hypertension, diabetes and cardiovascular diseases in later life, if proper nutrition is not provided.

SUMMARY

- Exclusive breastfeeding from birth until weaning is the optimal way to feed young infants.

- Continuing breastfeeding throughout weaning may reduce the risk of celiac disease, type 1 diabetes and wheat allergy.

- Weaning is recommended beginning around 6 months and avoiding certain high allergen foods before six months.

- However, recent evidence indicates that term infants should begin weaning by 6 months but not before 4 months (17 weeks).

- Potentially high allergen foods, such as egg, fish, milk used in food and cooking, cheese, yoghurt, wheat and other gluten containing cereals do not need to be delayed until a certain age (6–8 months).

- Preterm infants need special consideration and 5–8 months after their actual birth date is likely to be the best time to begin weaning. The majority may benefit from delaying until after 3 months after their estimated date of delivery to allow sufficient motor development.

  Monitor growth regularly and immunize your baby. You can monitor growth of your baby on the growth curves (IAP— 2007) based on affluent Indian children, given below (Agarwal et al, data).There are WHO growth charts based on international data; these are in use also.

Why NUTRITION for 5 to 10 years growth is very important?

- **Middle childhood—a slow, steady rate of physical growth. However, cognitive, emotional, and social development occur at a tremendous rate.**

- To achieve **optimal growth and development, children** need a variety of healthy **foods**.

- **Preparatory period for adolescence. Growth failure of this period** (undernutrition) will delay onset of pubescence. No catch up growth; further the peak height velocity will not be observed.

- Approximate growth in adolescence—Ht 25 cm in girls and 30 cm in boys; Wt 25–30 kg.

- **Lymphoid growth is maximum in this period (immunity).**

Table 6.2: DRI–30th November 2010

Age (year)	Protein (gm/day)	CHO (gm/day)	Calcium (mg)
4–8 Boys: 1200–2000 Girls: 1,200–1,800 cal	19	130	1000 mg (vitamin D = 600 IU)
9–11 Boys: 1600–2600 Girls: 1,400–2,200 cal	34	130	1300 mg (vitamin D = 600 IU)
14–18 Boys: 2000–3200 Girls: 1800–2400 cal	52 46	130 130	Same 1300/600
Sexual development			
Boys (>12 years)	60	3000 kcal/d	Boys–have lean body mass 2 times of girls—
Girls	46.0	2500 kcal/d	need more Fe, Ca and Zn

DRI—Dietary recommended intakes
CHO—Carbohydrates

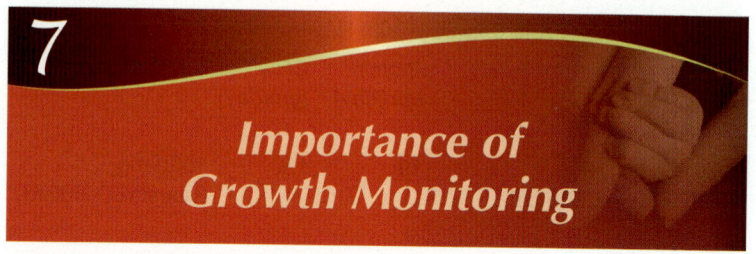

Importance of Growth Monitoring

The continuity of growth is important as this is the ultimate goal of good child health care and nutrition. Parents can also get some training and practice. For growth failure—no weight gain get alarmed. The growth curves are from Indian children (Agarwal et al. 1992, 1994, 2001—recommended by the Indian Academy of Pediatrics 2007).

We have also given WHO growth curves based on international data.

A separate growth curve for preterms is given.

MEASUREMENT OF HEIGHT, HEAD CIRCUMFERENCE AND WEIGHT

• *Length/height* is the best index of measuring linear growth (stature) as height reflects growth over a longer period than does weight.

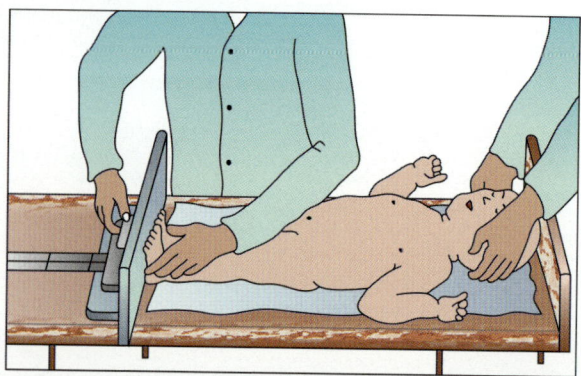

Fig. 7.1: Measuring length of an infant using infantometer (2 persons required for measurement)

- *Head circumference* can be used to assess brain growth in children mainly under-2 years, as during this period brain growth is very rapid (*at birth, the brain of the infant is 25% of the adult size. At the age of one year, the brain has grown to 75% of its adult size and to 80% by age of three, reaching 90% by age of seven*).

Measuring head circumference

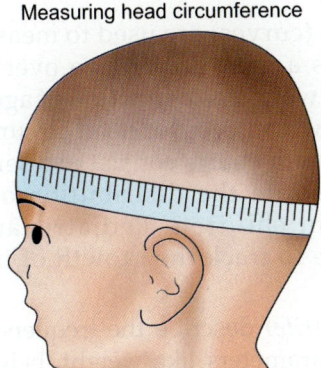

Proper positioning of measuring tape:
Widest circumference, avoiding ears

Fig. 7.2: Measurement of infant skull circumference using fiber glass tape

Weight-for-age is usually used to monitor growth. It is particularly useful in small infants who normally gain weight fast. Normal weight gain suggests that the infant is healthy and growing normally. Failure to gain weight normally is often the earliest sign of illness or malnutrition (i.e. undernutrition). Normally weight **doubles** by 5–6 months, **trebles** on first birth day and becomes **four times** of the birth weight at 2 years of age.

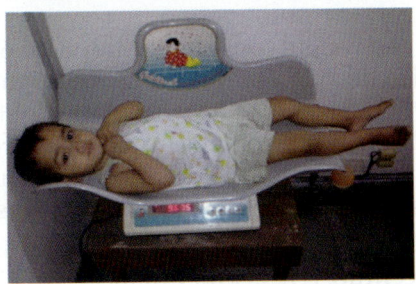

Fig. 7.3: Infant weight on electronic weighing scale

Growth monitoring is the regular measurement of a child's size in terms of length, weight and brain size as head circumference in order to document growth with age. The child's size measurements must then be plotted on a growth chart. This is extremely important as it can detect early changes in a child's growth. Both growing too slowly or too fast may indicate a health problem.

Growth charts (curves) are used to measure growth. The distance curve is a measure of size over time; it records length or height/weight as a function of age and gets higher with age (see growth curves for head circumference, height, and weight). Growth charts consist of a series of percentile curves that illustrate the distribution of selected body measurements in children. Pediatricians, nurses, and parents use these to track the growth of infants, children, and adolescents.

Percentiles (centile) describe the frequency distribution of anthropometric parameters like weight, height, skull circumference, etc. 50th percentile is the average (median) line for the given population, describes the percent of children expected to be on or below that line and, e.g. 50th centile means that 49% of the observations are below and 50% above that observation. A child's growth parameters may be on the centile line or between two centile lines. **Conventionally, for all parameters, 3rd and 97th percentiles are the lowest and highest 94% of observations having normal children.**

- *Any child with parameters below or above these limits or those who cross percentiles after 2 years of age needs careful evaluation.*

- *Examples:*
  a. If height and weight consistently are on the 60th percentile line until a child is 5 years old, then the height has dropped to the 30th percentile at age of 6, that might indicate that there is a growth problem (catch down retardation of growth) because the child is not following his or her previous growth pattern—this indicates disease.
  b. Boy with height in 40th percentile and weight in the 85th percentile. (He is taller than 40% of kids of his age, but weighs more than 85% of kids of his age.) There

might be a health problem (overweight/obesity). On the other hand, if he is in the 85th percentile for height and weight and follows that pattern consistently over time, that usually means that he is a normal child, just larger than average.

The growth curves recommended by the Indian Academy of Pediatrics in 2007 Agarwal *et al* 1992, 1994, 2001 are to be followed for regular growth assessment.

Monitoring Height—Weight by Parents/Family Members

1. Growth monitoring by a *trainable* family member who has learnt from a health worker is an ideal approach for weight recordings with increasing age. It will help to assess that child is gaining weight—**good health** OR if there is loss in weight on monthly recordings—*warning sign poor feeding or illness.*

2. Length/height measurements in infancy and early childhood are very difficult, however may serve as an approximate/ close estimates. Parents can measure on a flat hard smooth surface, mark the length head to foot, then measure with fibre glass tape.

Limitations: Wrong measurement of the weight or height by untrained or half-trained hands can miss growth faltering. Still we must train family to record weight on monthly intervals in first 12 months; on alternate months in 2nd year and 3 monthly up to the age of 5–6 years.

Fortunately, infants and children are visiting the health centers for immunizations, this is the unique opportunity to record—length, head circumference and weight by trained hands and calibrated tools. These values be plotted on a growth curve to compare with the early date, if increment is following the growth percentile curve *Good*—if not, *worry*.

Physical Growth in Children

Anthropometric measures of normal full term newborn:

Birth weight: 2.7–4.6 kg

Length: 50 cm (around)

Head circumference: 34–35 cm

Weight Gain

Neonates generally lose 5–8% (maximum being 10%) weight during first 2–3 days of life, which is regained by the 10th day. Average daily weight gain during—

First 3 months: 30 gm

3–6 months: 20 gm (birth weight doubles by 5–6 months of age)

6–9 months: 15 gm

9–12 months: 12 gm (birth weight triples by first birthday).

1–3 years: 8 gm (around 3 kg/year). Birth weight quadruples by 2 years of age.

4–6 years: 6 gm (around 2 kg/year); this rate of gain continues till the onset of puberty.

Length/Height Gain (Height Velocity)

Birth to 3 months: 3.5 cm/month

3–6 months: 2.0 cm/month

6–9 months: 1.5 cm/month

9–12 months: 1.2 cm/month

1–3 years: 1.0 cm/month

4–6 years: 5 cm/year (at 4 years = 100 cm; double of birth length)

Gain in Length

- During 1st year of life: 25 cm
- During 2nd year of life: 12.5 cm
- During 3rd year of life: 7.5–10 cm
- 7 cm/year at 3–4 yrs
- 6 cm/year at 5–6 yrs
- 5 cm/year till puberty
- In immediate prepubertal period, growth velocity slows down before the pubertal spurt begins (adenarche).

Abnormal Growth

- < 7 cm/year for < 4yr age
- < 6 cm/year for 4–6 yrs
- < 4.5 cm/year for 6 yrs–onset of puberty

Key Notes

- Head circumference represents brain growth—it is very rapid during first 12 months.
- Length represents main body growth.
- Weight represents current nutritional status, fall or rapid rise are ALARMING signs and suggest disease.

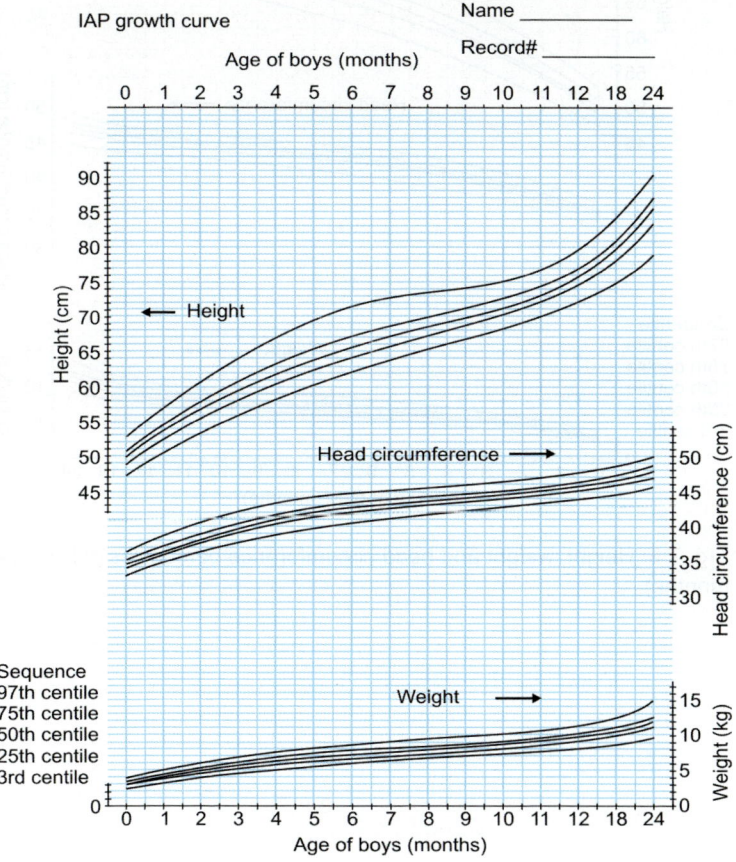

Fig. 7.4: Height, weight and head circumference percentiles boys (0–24 months)

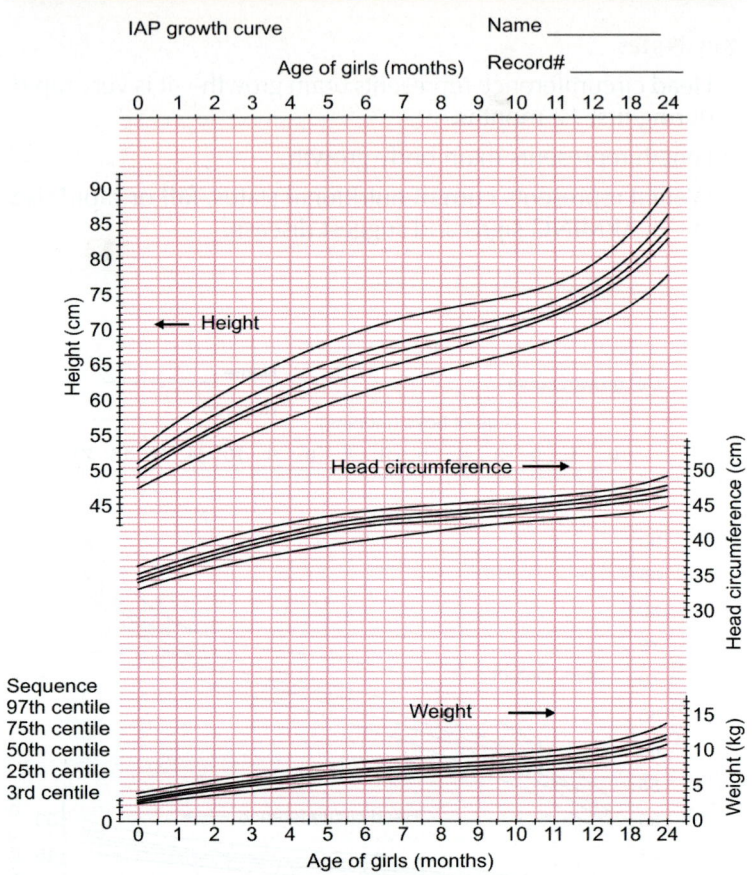

Fig. 7.5: Height, weight and head circumference percentiles girls (0–24 months)

Name _____

Record# _____

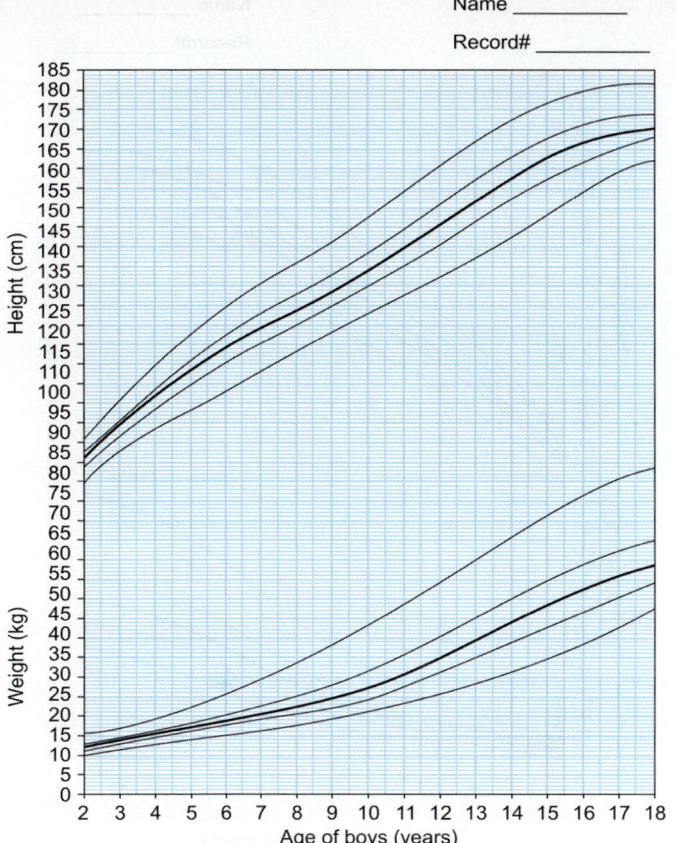

Fig. 7.6: Height, weight percentiles boys (2–18 years)

Name _____

Record# _____

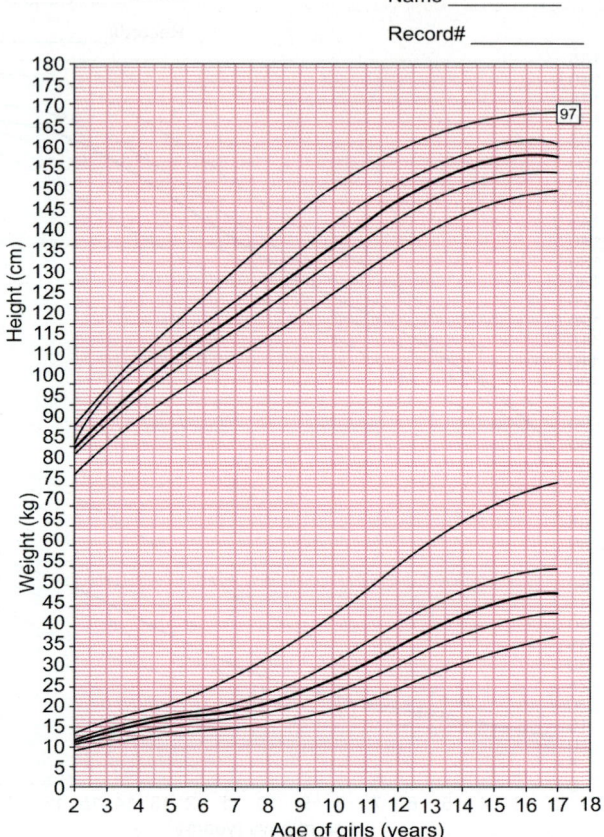

Fig. 7.7: Height, weight, percentiles girls (2–17 years)

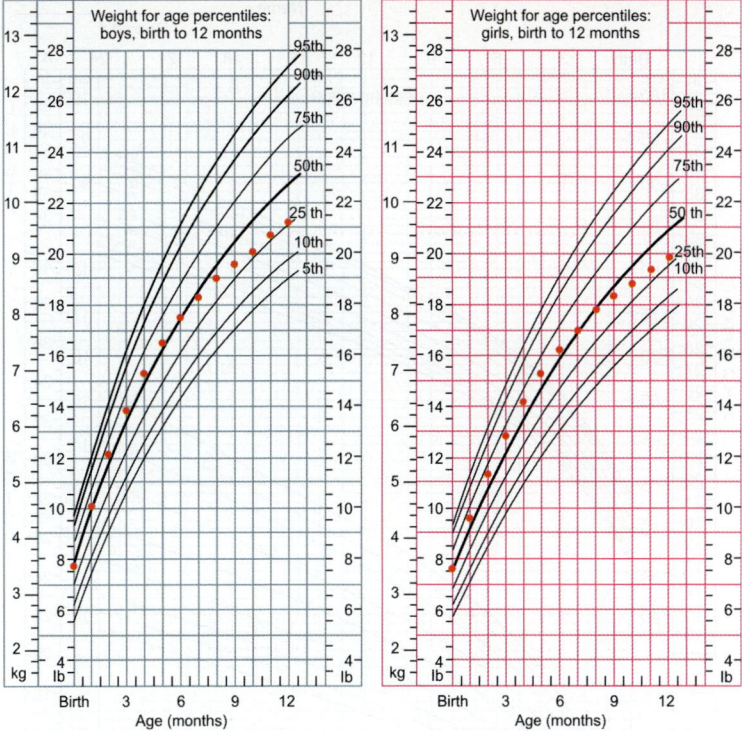

Sources:

– **Base chart**—CDC Growth Charts: United States, Published May 30,2000

Graphic by *kellymom.com,* **2004**

– **Breastfed baby data points**—WHO Working Group on Infant Growth. An Evaluation of Infant Growth a summary of analyses performed in preparation for the WHO Expert Committee on Physical Status: the use and interpretation of anthropometry. (WHO/NUT/94.8). Geneva: World Health Organization, 1994, p.21

Fig. 7.8: Average growth patterns of breastfed infants. The red points plotted on the CDG growth charts represent the average weight-for-age for a small set of infant boys and girls who were breastfed for at least 12 months

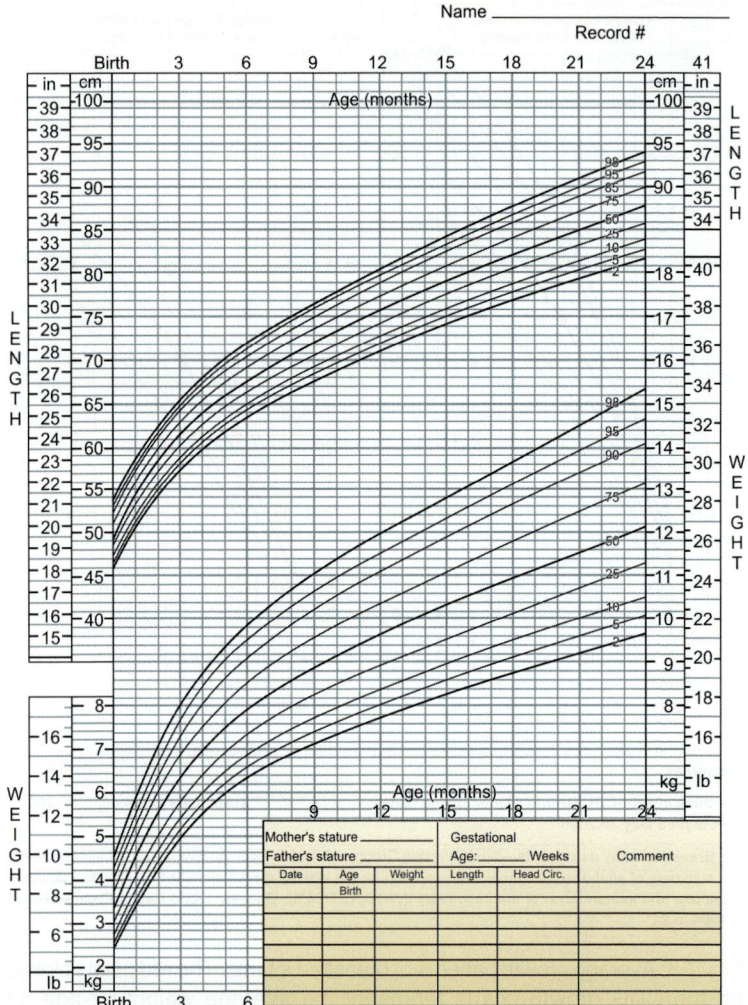

Published by the Centers for Disease Control and Prevention, November 1, 2009

Sources: WHO Child Growth Standards (http://www.who.int/childgrowth/en)

Fig. 7.9: Length-for-age and weight-for-age percentiles, birth to 24 months for boys. (WHO growth curves)

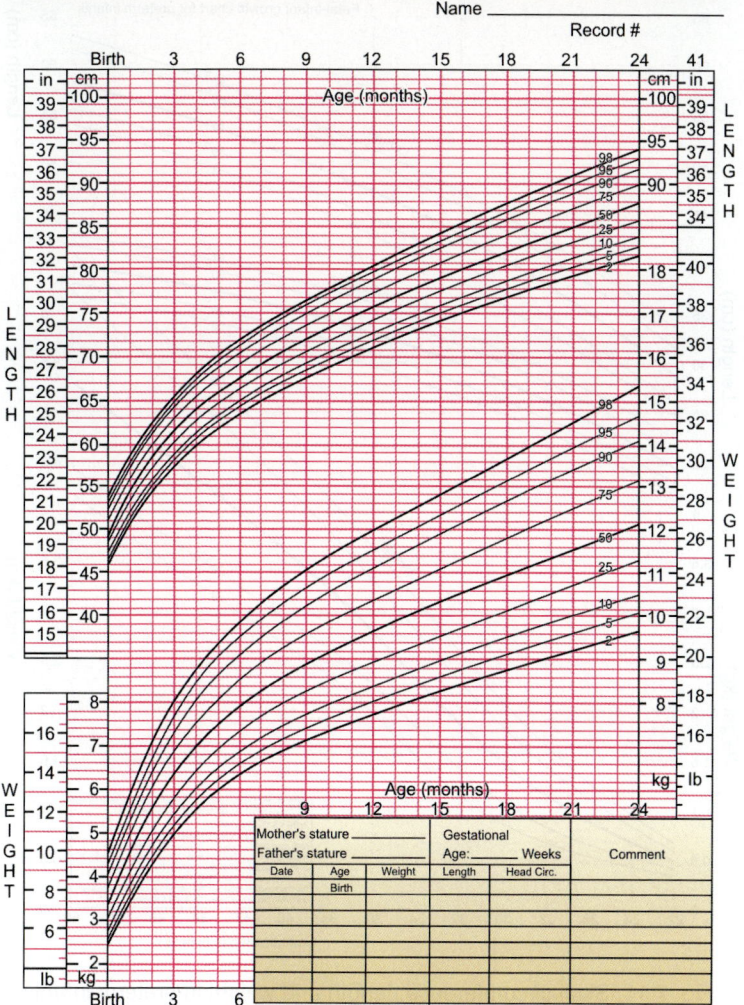

Published by the Centers for Disease Control and Prevention, November 1, 2009

Sources: WHO Child Growth Standards (http://www.who.int/childgrowth/en)

Fig. 7.10: Length-for-age and weight-for-age percentiles, birth to 24 months for girls. (WHO growth curves)

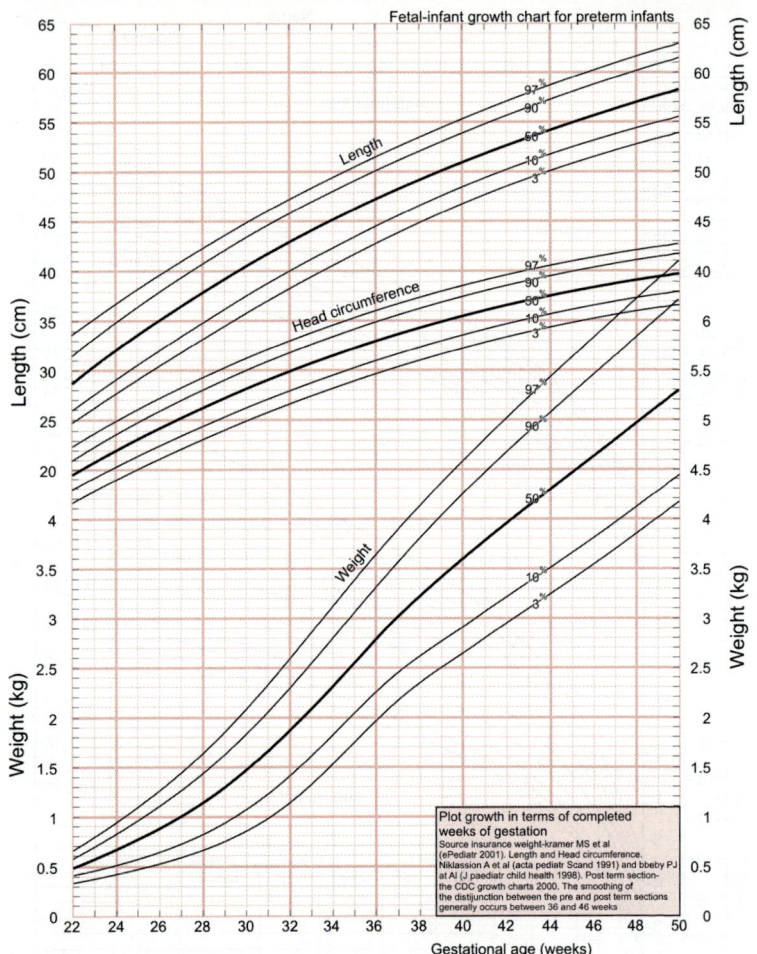

Fig. 7.11: Skull circumference, length and weight in preterm infants

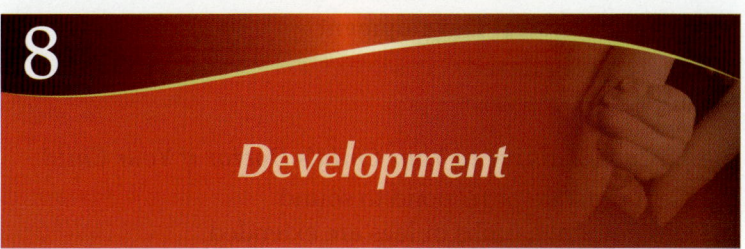

8

Development

Parents are always eager to observe and compare developmental milestones. This is discussed in detail here.

Table 8.1: Primitive reflexes

Reflexes	Appearance	Disappearance
Moro	Birth	4 months
Hand grasp	Birth	3 months
Atonic neck reflex	2 weeks	6 months
Protective equilibrium	4–6 months	Persists voluntarily
Head righting	4–6 months	–do–
Parachute	8–9 months	–do–

Developmental Red Flags

Primitive reflexes persisting past 6 months.
No head control by 3 months.
Fisting beyond 3 months.
Mouthing of objects beyond 6–8 months.

Newborn

Social and Emotional
- Fixates on face in preference to other objects
  Language/communication
- Startles or widens eyes to sound
- Shows variation in crying

Cognitive (Learning, Thinking, Problem-Solving)
- Can fixate on face at 8–15 inches
- Visual acuity: 20/400

Movement/Physical Development

- Arms and leg flexed
- Poor head control

Act Early by Talking to Your Child's Doctor if Your Child

- Does not fixate or respond to sound
- Does not move limbs or legs are extended

IMPORTANT MILESTONES

Most Babies can Do at 2 Months of Age

Social and Emotional

- Begins to smile at people
- Can briefly calm himself (may bring hands to mouth and suck on hand)
- Tries to look at parent

Language/Communication

- Coos, makes gurgling sounds
- Turns head toward sounds

Cognitive (Learning, Thinking, Problem-Solving)

- Pays attention to faces
- Begins to follow things with eyes and recognize people at a distance
- Begins to act bored (cries, fussy) if activity does not change

Movement/Physical Development

- Can hold head up and begins to push up when lying on tummy
- Makes smoother movements with arms and legs

Act Early by Talking to Your Child's Doctor if Your Child

- Does not respond to loud sounds
- Does not watch things as they move
- Does not smile at people
- Does not bring hands to mouth
- Cannot hold head up when pushing up when on tummy.

Most Babies can Do at 4 Months of Age

Social and Emotional

- Smiles spontaneously, especially at people (Fig. 8.1)
- Likes to play with people and might cry when playing stops
- Copies some movements and facial expressions, like smiling or frowning

Language/Communication

- Begins to babble
- Babbles with expression and copies sounds he hears
- Cries in different ways to show hunger, pain, or being tired

Cognitive (Learning, Thinking, Problem-Solving)

- Lets you know if she/he is happy or sad
- Responds to affection
- Reaches for toy with one hand
- Uses hands and eyes together, such as seeing a toy and reaching for it
- Follows moving things with eyes from side to side
- Watches faces closely
- Recognizes familiar people and things at a distance

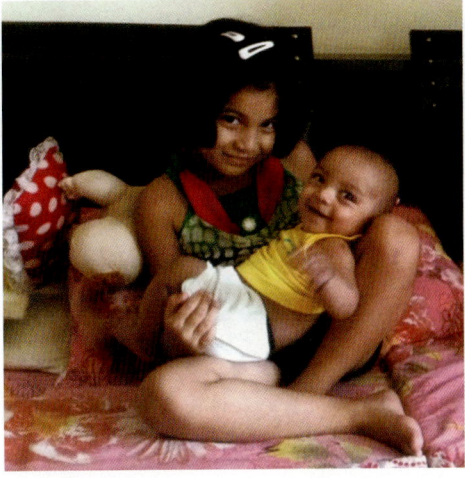

Fig. 8.1: Sister playing with younger brother, educative acts

Movement/Physical Development

- Holds head steady, unsupported (Fig. 8.2)
- Pushes down on legs when feet are on a hard surface
- May be able to roll over from tummy to back
- Can hold a toy and shake it and swing at dangling toys
- Brings hands to mouth
- When lying on stomach, pushes up to elbows

Act Early by Talking to Your Child's Doctor if Your Child

- Does not watch things as they move
- Does not smile at people
- Cannot hold head steady
- Does not coo or make sounds
- Does not bring things to mouth
- Does not push down with legs when feet are placed on a hard surface
- Has trouble moving one or both eyes in all directions.

Most Babies can Do at 6 Months of Age

Social and Emotional

- Knows familiar faces and begins to know if someone is a stranger
- Likes to play with others, especially parents
- Responds to other people's emotions and often seems happy
- Likes to look at self in a mirror

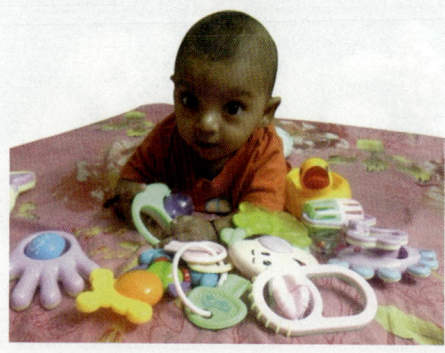

Fig. 8.2: Baby holding head steady, unsupported

Language/Communication

- Responds to sounds by making sounds
- Strings vowels together when babbling ("ah", "eh", "oh") and likes taking turns with parent while making sounds
- Responds to own name
- Makes sounds to show joy and displeasure
- Begins to say consonant sounds (jabbering with "m", "b")

Cognitive (Learning, Thinking, Problem-Solving)

- Looks around at things nearby
- Brings things to mouth
- Shows curiosity about things and tries to get things that are out of reach
- Begins to pass things from one hand to the other

Movement/Physical Development

- Rolls over in both directions (front-to-back, back-to-front)
- Begins to sit without support
- When standing, supports weight on legs and might bounce
- Rocks back and forth, sometimes crawling backward before moving forward (Fig. 8.3).

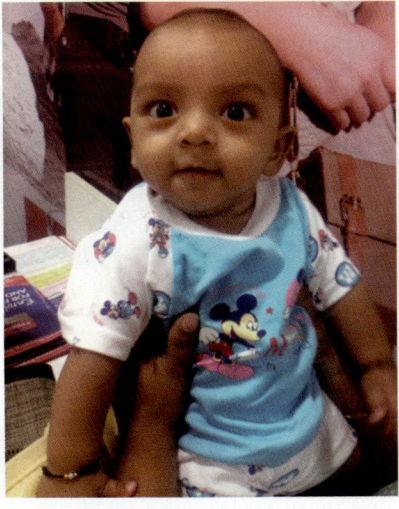

Fig. 8.3: Held standing, supports weight on legs

Act Early by Talking to Your Child's Doctor if Your Child

- Does not try to get things that are in reach
- Shows no affection for caregivers
- Does not respond to sounds around him
- Has difficulty getting things to mouth
- Does not make vowel sounds ("ah", "eh", "oh")
- Does not roll over in either direction
- Does not laugh or make squealing sounds
- Seems very stiff, with tight muscles
- Seems very floppy, like a rag doll

Most Babies can Do at 9 Months of Age

Social and Emotional

- May be afraid of strangers
- May be clingy with familiar adults
- Has favorite toys

Language/Communication

- Understands "no"
- Makes a lot of different sounds like "mama mama" and "babababba"
- Copies sounds and gestures of others
- Uses fingers to point at things (Fig. 8.4)

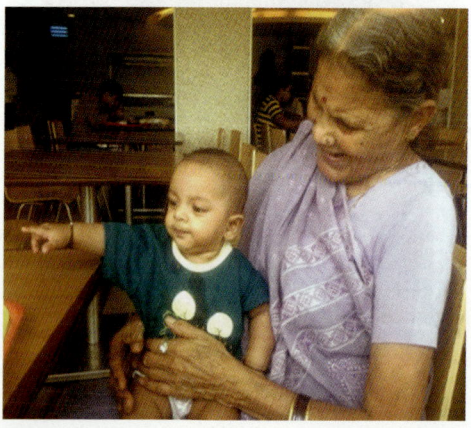

Fig. 8.4: Infant with grandmother, pointing finger to an object

Cognitive (Learning, Thinking, Problem-Solving)
- Watches the path of something as it falls
- Looks for things he sees you hide
- Plays peek-a-boo
- Puts things in mouth
- Moves things smoothly from one hand to the other
- Picks up things between thumb and index finger (Pincer grasp)

Movement/Physical Development
- Stands, holding on
- Can get into sitting position
- Sits without support
- Pulls to stand
- Crawls

Act Early by Talking to Your Child's Doctor if Your Child
- Does not bear weight on legs with support
- Does not sit with help
- Does not babble ("mama", "baba", "dada")
- Does not play any games involving back-and-forth play
- Does not respond to own name
- Does not seem to recognize familiar people
- Does not look where you point
- Does not transfer toys from one hand to the other

Most Children can Do at 1 Year of Age

Social and Emotional
- Is shy or nervous with strangers
- Cries when mom or dad leaves
- Has favorite things and people
- Shows fear in some situations
- Hands you a book when he wants to hear a story
- Repeats sounds or actions to get attention
- Puts out arm or leg to help with dressing
- Plays games such as "peek-a-boo" and "pat-a-cake"

Language/Communication

- Responds to simple spoken requests
- Uses simple gestures, like shaking head "no" or waving "bye-bye"
- Makes sounds with changes in tone (sounds more like speech)
- Says "mama" and "dada" and exclamations like "uh-oh!"
- Tries to say words which you say

Cognitive (Learning, Thinking, Problem-Solving)

- Explores things in different ways, like shaking, banging, throwing
- Finds hidden things easily
- Looks at the right picture or thing when it is named
- Copies gestures
- Starts to use things correctly; for example, drinks from a cup, brushes hair
- Bangs two things together
- Puts things in a container, takes things out of a container
- Lets things go without help
- Pokes with index (pointer) finger
- Follows simple directions like "pick up the toy"

Movement/Physical Development

- Gets to a sitting position without help
- Pulls up to stand, walks holding on to furniture ("cruising")
- May take a few steps without holding on
- May stand alone

Act Early by Talking to Your Child's Doctor if Your Child

- Does not crawl
- Cannot stand when supported
- Does not search for things that she sees you hide
- Does not say single words like "mama" or "dada"
- Does not learn gestures like waving or shaking head
- Does not point to things
- Loses skills he once had

- By 15 months, your child is able to walk alone with feet wide apart and arms held high to maintain balance. Also pushes tricycle (Fig. 8.5).

Most Babies can Do at 18 Months of Age

Social and Emotional

- Likes to hand things to others as play
- May have temper tantrums
- May be afraid of strangers
- Shows affection to familiar people
- Plays simple pretend, such as feeding a doll
- May cling to caregivers in new situations
- Points to show others something interesting
- Explores alone but with parent close by

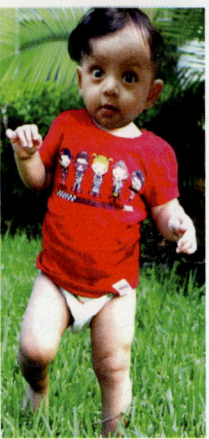

Fig. 8.5: 15 months old child walks with wide feet and hands held high for balance

Language/Communication

Says several single words
- Says and shakes head "no"
- Points to show someone what he wants

Cognitive (Learning, Thinking, Problem-Solving)

- Knows what ordinary things are for; for example, telephone, brush, spoon
- Points to get the attention of others
- Shows interest in a doll or stuffed animal by pretending to feed
- Points to one's body part
- Scribbles on his own
- Can follow 1-step verbal commands without any gestures; for example, sits when you say "sit down"

Movement/Physical Development

- Walks alone
- May walk up steps and run
- Pulls toys while walking
- Can help undress herself

- Drinks from a cup
- Eats with a spoon

Act Early by Talking to Your Child's Doctor if Your Child

- Does not point to show things to others
- Cannot walk
- Does not know what familiar things are for
- Does not copy others
- Does not gain new words
- Does not have at least 6 words
- Does not notice or mind when a caregiver leaves or returns
- Loses skills he once had

Most Babies can Do at 2 Years of Age

Social and Emotional

- Copies others, especially adults and older children
- Gets excited when with other children
- Shows more and more independence
- Shows defiant behavior (doing what he has been told not to)
- Plays mainly beside other children, but is beginning to include other children, such as in chase games

Language/Communication

- Points to things or pictures when they are named
- Knows names of familiar people and body parts
- Says sentences with 2 to 4 words
- Follows simple instructions
- Repeats words overheard in conversation
- Points to things in a book

Cognitive (Learning, Thinking, Problem-Solving)

- Finds things even when hidden under two or three covers
- Begins to sort shapes and colors
- Completes sentences and rhymes in familiar books
- Plays simple make-believe games
- Builds towers of 4 or more blocks
- Might use one hand more than the other

- Follows two-step instructions such as "pick up your shoes and put them in the closet."
- Names items in a picture book such as a cat, bird, or dog (Fig. 8.6)

Movement/Physical Development

- Stands on tiptoe
- Kicks a ball
- Begins to run
- Climbs onto and down from furniture without help
- Walks up- and downstairs holding on
- Throws ball overhand
- Makes or copies straight lines and circles

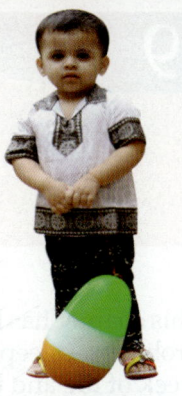

Fig. 8.6: Child playing with a baloon

Act Early by Talking to Your Child's Doctor if Your Child

- Does not use 2-word phrases (for example, "drink milk")
- Does not know what to do with common things, like a brush, phone, fork, spoon
- Does not copy actions and words
- Does not follow simple instructions
- Does not walk steadily
- Loses skills she/he once had

Key Notes
- Baby failing to achieve expected for age milestones warns of abnormalities in growth and brain development.
- Test hearing and vision.

9

Common Baby Care Points

This chapter has key messages as how to solve small childhood problems—sleep, cry, colic, number of stools, jaundice in first week of life and breast enlargement.

A. SLEEP

Expect your newborn baby to be asleep for up to 18 hours over the course of 24 hours in his first few weeks. But he would not sleep for more than three hours or four hours at a time, day or night.

This is a necessary phase for your baby and it would not last long.

Baby's sleep cycles are short as he will spend more time in rapid eye movement (REM) sleep, which is a light, easily disturbed sleep. This is necessary for the changes that are happening in his brain.

6–8 weeks old baby will sleep for shorter spells during the day and longer periods at night. But he will still wake up to feed during the night. He will have more deep, non-REM sleep and less light sleep.

After 8 weeks baby may sleep through night. But it is more likely that your nights will be interrupted for at least the first few months. We have tried giving bath in the evening followed by massage; this has encouraged night sleep.

Your baby can develop good sleep habits from as early as six weeks. Here are a few tactics you can use to help your baby to settle.

Recognize the Signs that Mean He is Tired

During your baby's first three months, learn the signs that he is sleepy, such as if he:

• Rubs his eyes

- Flicks his ear with his hand
- Develops faint, dark circles under his eyes
- Whines and cries at the slightest provocation
- Stares blankly into space
- Yawns and stretches a lot
- Loses interest in people and toys
- Becomes quiet and still

He may also turn his face away from moving objects or people, or bury his face in your chest.

If you spot these or any other signs of sleepiness, try putting him down in his cot. You will soon develop baby's daily rhythms and patterns, and know instinctively when he is ready for sleep.

Teach Him the Difference Between Night and Day

From the 2nd week in the daytime, when he is alert, try:
- Change his clothes when he wakes to signal the start of a new day
- Play/talk with him as much as you can
- Make daytime feeds social. Chat and sing during feeding
- Keep the house and his room light and bright
- Let him hear everyday noises, such as the radio, fan, or washing machine
- Wake him gently if he sleeps during a feed

At Night-Time

- Stay quiet when you feed him
- Keep lights and noise low, and do not talk to him too much
- Change him into his pajamas to signal the end of the day

All this should help your baby to start understand that night time is for sleeping.

Give Him a Chance to Fall Asleep on His Own

When your baby's between 6 and 8 weeks old, you can teach him how to fall asleep. Many babies hold blanket, or toy or like to hear some music and go to sleep. Put him down when he is sleepy, but still awake. Stay with him if you wish, but be prepared to do the same everytime he wakes at night. You will need to adopt the same strategy every night.

At 3 months, most babies sleep a total of 15 hours a day, including night time sleep and naps.

By the age of 4 months or so, babies have started to develop more of a regular sleep/wake pattern and have dropped most of their night feeds.

At some point between 4 and 6 months, most babies are capable of sleeping through the night (for 8 to 12 hours).

B. CRYING

Babies cry. It is how they communicate—
* Hunger
* Pain
* Fear
* A need for sleep
* A dirty diaper
* Wants to be held
* Wants burping
* Tummy trouble
* Wants security, play, etc.

C. COLIC

Baby colic (also known as **infantile colic**) is a condition in which an otherwise healthy baby cries or displays symptoms of distress (cramping, moaning, etc.) frequently and for extended periods, without any discernible reason. The condition typically appears within the first month of life and often disappears rather suddenly, before the baby is three to four months old, but can last up to one year. Another study concluded that babies who are not breastfed are almost twice as likely to have colic. *Epidemiology suggests that chocolate, cabbage, onions, and cow's milk are among the foods that a lactating mother may need to avoid.*

The crying often increases during a specific period of the day, particularly the early evening.

It is well established that there are a variety of causes of colic symptoms, the most common of which includes stomach gas (possibly due to poor burping or milk flow issues), intestinal gas (pocketed in the intestinal tract), neurological overload (the overwhelmed and over stimulated baby that becomes exhausted) and even a muscular type of colic (perhaps due to muscle spasm and birth trauma). A gastrointestinal (GI) theory of colic seems logical because fussy babies often grunt/pass gas/double-up/cry after eating. They improve with stomach pressure, warmth or massage; may improve with pain medication. However, 85–90% of colicky babies have no evidence of serious gut abnormality.

Colic could be due to transient lactase deficiency, temporary lactose intolerance in young infants.

D. NUMBER OF STOOLS PER DAY

Normally "newborns" in early months can pass 8–10 soft yellow stools in a day or may pass once in 5–6 days.

E. JAUNDICE IN FIRST WEEK (PHYSIOLOGICAL JAUNDICE)

i. *Physiological (normal) jaundice:* Occurring in most newborns, this mild jaundice is due to the immaturity of the baby's liver, which leads to a slow processing of bilirubin. It generally appears at 2 to 4 days of age and disappears by 1 to 2 weeks of age.

ii. *Jaundice of prematurity:* Occurs frequently in premature babies since they are even less ready to excrete bilirubin effectively. Jaundice in premature baby needs to be treated at a lower bilirubin level than in full term babies in order to avoid serious neurological and hearing complications.

iii. *Breast milk jaundice:* In 1–2% of breastfed babies, jaundice may be caused by substances produced in their mother's breast milk that can cause the bilirubin level to rise. These can prevent the excretion of bilirubin through the intestines. It starts after the first 3 to 5 days and slowly improves over 3 to 12 weeks.

F. NEONATAL BREAST ENLARGEMENT

It is a normal response to falling levels of maternal estrogen at the end of pregnancy, which trigger the release of prolactin from the newborn's pituitary. Neonatal breast enlargement is common (seen in approximately 70% of neonates), and is independent of the sex of the baby. It usually occurs in the first week of life and resolves within a few weeks. The enlarged breast may discharge liquid; this usually resolves without treatment over a period of a few weeks. Squeezing the breast to facilitate the discharge may lead to irritation, further enlargement, persistence of the hypertrophied tissue, or, in rare cases, infection (mastitis or abscess).

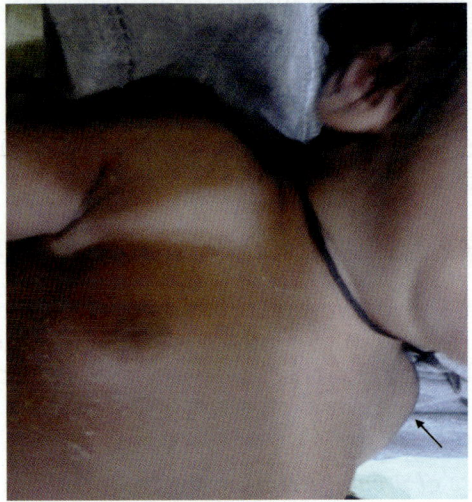

Fig. 9.1: Neonatal breast enlargement

G. HYPOGLYCEMIA

Hypoglycemia (reduced blood sugar in baby's blood) is the most common metabolic problem in neonates. Newborn may present with severe central nervous system (CNS) and cardio-pulmonary disturbances. The most common clinical manifestations can include altered level of consciousness, *seizure*, vomiting, unresponsiveness, and lethargy. Sustained hypoglycemia in newborn has a major impact on normal brain development and function (causing brain damage that may permanently impair neurologic development).

The WHO directive of strict breastfeeding immediately after birth should not be rigidly followed for mothers after caesarian delivery or those who have not started lactating especially in the case of first child birth or other co-existing pregnancy complications.

In case of our grand child (first child + caesarian delivery) AIIMS, New Delhi, after some hours (late evening), Prof Vinod K Paul visited and took away the supplemental formula, despite the mother (a qualified obstetrician) informing about lactation not being established and the baby's poor sucking. After repeated requests for repeat assessment regarding the neonate's feeding, the team failed to make a timely diagnosis of hypoglycemia and the baby suffered hypoglycemic seizures with cardiac arrest. Till this day and for the rest of his life, the child has to fight the consequences of permanent brain damage due to these events. The message is to individualize treatment and avoid one of the important preventable cause of permanent brain injury. The message for pediatricians is to consider a mother's concerns and for moms to feed the baby timely during the period lactation has not established.

H. HYPOCALCEMIA

Hypocalcemia is a condition in which there is too little calcium in a baby's blood. A common form of hypocalcemia in babies is called neonatal hypocalcemia. This condition may occur at different times for different reasons:

- Early hypocalcemia occurs in the first three days of life.
- Late hypocalcemia develops between the fifth to tenth day of life, usually after several days of formula feedings.

Symptoms of hypocalcemia may not be obvious in newborn babies. The following are the most common symptoms of hypocalcemia:

- Irritability
- Muscle twitches
- Jitteriness
- Tremors
- Poor feeding
- Lethargy
- Seizures

This is common in babies of mothers who have not taken vitamin D and calcium regularly in pregnancy.

Vaginal Bleeding

Newborn girls have been exposed to many hormones in the uterus. Among other things, these hormones may have:

- made the outside of the vagina ("labia majora" and the "clitoris") a little swollen and prominent.
- caused a thick, milky discharge in the vagina.

Most dramatically, at 2 or 3 days of age, your daughter may have a little bit of bleeding from her vagina. This is perfectly normal—it is caused by the withdrawal of the hormones she was exposed to in the womb. It will be her first and last menstrual period for another decade or so.

Key Notes

- Mother/baby care giver should learn about sleep pattern, crying causes, and colic.
- Breast fed baby may pass 8–10 stools—soft and yellow or once in 5–6 days.
- JAUNDICE in first hours or day is serious—consult the pediatrician. Jaundice pigment deposits in brain and causes permanent damage.
- Low blood sugar level and calcium level can cause seizures (fit-jerky movements)—both deficiencies can damage brain.
- Breast enlargement and vaginal bleeding are temporary, due to maternal hormones.

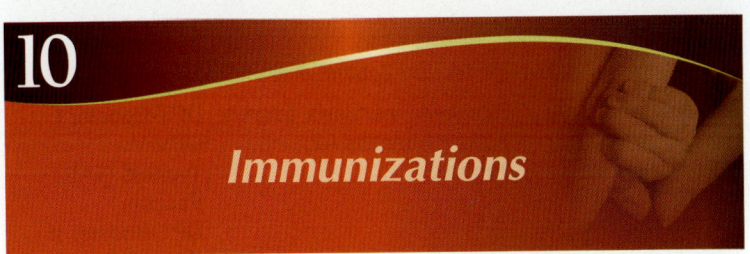

Immunizations

This is the best technology to prevent diseases and keep our children healthy. Some vaccines are costly, freely discuss with your doctor to manage within pocket.

IMMUNIZATION SCHEDULE

Currently available vaccines are the high level technological achievements reaching our door steps. Some are costly, thus it is for the family to plan that essential vaccines reach their child within the budget.

Age of immunization	Protection against disease	Vaccine
At birth	Hepatitis B, polio, tuberculosis	Hep B vaccine-I OPV-zero dose BCG
4–6 weeks	Hepatitis B, diphtheria, pertussis, tetanus	Hep B vaccine-II DPT-I
6 weeks	Polio, *H. influenzae* (brain fever)	OPV-I HiB-I
10 weeks	Diphtheria, pertussis, tetanus, polio, *H. influenzae* (brain fever)	DPT-II OPV-II HiB-II
14 weeks	Diphtheria, pertussis, tetanus, polio, *H. influenzae* (brain fever)	DPT-III OPV-III HiB-III
6 months	Hepatitis B	Hep B vaccine-III
9 months	Measles and polio	Measles vaccine OPV-IV
15 months	Chicken pox (ideally give twice) + hepatitis A	Varicella vaccine*
15–18 months	Mumps, measles and rubella	MMR-I

*Varicella and MMR should not be administered together.

(contd.)

(contd.)

Age of immunization	Protection against disease	Vaccine
18–24 months	Diphtheria, pertussis, tetanus, polio + hepatitis A2	DPT-Booster I OPV-V
24 months	Typhoid	Typhoid (TAB) Vaccine DPT-Booster II OPV-VI MMR-II-Booster is recommended
4½–5 years	Diphtheria, pertussis and tetanus, polio, mumps, measles and rubella chicken pox (2)	• *Note BCG protects against severity of tuberculosis especially meningitis; acellular pertussis vaccine gives lower immune response but does not cause fever*

POINTS TO REMEMBER

• Combination vaccines are available for DPT + Hib vaccine (quadrivalent vaccine) and DPT + hepatitis B + Hib vaccine (pentavalent vaccine). These can be used to decrease the number of pricks being given to the baby and to decrease the number of clinic visits.

• OPV must be given to children less than 5 years of age at the time of each supplementary immunization activity, i.e. pulse polio schemes.

• In view of poor water/food quality, the hepatitis A 2 shots within 6 months be given among essential vaccines.

CONTINUATION OF VACCINATION AFTER 5 YEARS OF AGE

• T.T vaccination against tetanus is recommended at every five year interval.

• Typhoid vaccination against typhoid infection is recommended at every three year interval.

• MMR 2nd dose

• Chicken pox second dose

OTHER RECOMMENDED VACCINES

These vaccines can be administered along with the schedule given above, under guidance of your **pediatrician**. The vaccines are not yet part of vaccination schedule of Indian Government, but are recommended by the Indian Academy of Pediatrics.

1. Pneumococcal conjugate vaccine against pneumococcal pneumonia—three primary doses at 6, 10, and 14 weeks, followed by a booster at 15–18 months (*costly*).
2. Rotavirus vaccine against infant diarrhea due to rotavirus—two doses 4 weeks apart usually given at 6 weeks and 10 weeks (*costly*).
3. Hepatitis A vaccine against hepatitis A jaundice—it is given after age of 12 months, i.e. 1 year of age; two doses at 6 months interval (*we think it is essential to protect from infective hepatitis*).
4. TIV or influenza vaccine against influenza virus infections—two doses after 6 months of age at 4 week interval, then yearly.
5. Meningococcal polysaccharide A and C vaccine against meningococcal infections is recommended in immuno-compromised children, splenectomy or when there is disease outbreak in community—single dose above age of one year.
6. HPV vaccine against HPV infections known to cause cervical cancer—it is as yet given to girls above age of 10 years; three doses; 0, 1 month and 6 months.

Key Notes

- Vaccines have successfully controlled deadly early childhood diseases.
- It is important to get your child immunized for all essential vaccines and choose optional vaccines as per budget.

Index

Reader's Notes

Reader's Notes